ANTENATAL
CARE

Dr. Miriam Stoppard

ANTENATAL CARE

DORLING KINDERSLEY
London • New York • Sydney • Moscow

HEALTHCARE

A DORLING KINDERSLEY BOOK

DESIGN AND EDITORIAL Edward Kinsey and Jacqueline Jackson

SENIOR MANAGING ART EDITOR Lynne Brown
MANAGING EDITOR Jemima Dunne

SENIOR ART EDITOR Karen Ward
SENIOR EDITOR Penny Warren

PRODUCTION Antony Heller

First published in Great Britain in 1998 by
Dorling Kindersley Limited, 9 Henrietta Street,
Covent Garden, London WC2E 8PS

Visit us on the World Wide Web at http://www.dk.com

Material in this publication was previously published by
Dorling Kindersley in *Conception, Pregnancy and Birth*
by Dr. Miriam Stoppard.

A CIP catalogue record for this book is available
from the British Library.

ISBN 0-7513-0547-2

Reproduced by Colourscan, Singapore and IGS, Radstock, Avon
Printed in Hong Kong by Wing King Tong

CONTENTS

INTRODUCTION 6

INTRODUCTION

After receiving the exciting news that you are pregnant, you'll have lots to think about and prepare: what kind of birth do I want – in hospital or at home, with medical management or as natural as possible? What are the options for pain relief? The choices are yours but it's worth looking into the various childbirth philosophies. You then need to discuss your ideas fully with your partner, doctor and midwife. When you have decided, it's a good idea to write a birth plan so that everyone is aware of your preferences.

Attending all your antenatal check-ups is vital to protect the well-being of both you and your baby. At the antenatal clinic, you'll have routine tests that are designed to spot any problems and treat them promptly if necessary. Special tests such as ultrasound scans and amniocentesis are offered to enable doctors to investigate the baby's health in more detail. Regular antenatal care can provide reassurance, and the chance to discuss issues that you may be concerned about.

YOUR DEVELOPING BABY

For you, early pregnancy means that high levels of pregnancy hormones bring on nausea or sickness, the need to go the lavatory more often and breast tenderness.

As your pregnancy becomes established, you will probably be keen to understand the developmental stages of your unborn baby and how you can provide the best chance of good health. This means taking action such as giving up smoking and avoiding alcohol and trying to maintain a balanced diet. Keeping fit and supple in pregnancy enables your body to cope better with the extra weight; you'll also find it easier to recover from the delivery.

The majority of women have normal pregnancies but for those with existing medical conditions or an unexpected problem such as high blood pressure, it can be a very worrying time. However, with careful monitoring and treatment, most pregnancies have a successful outcome.

1

YOUR PREGNANCY TIMETABLE

Discovering that you are pregnant for the first time can be one of the most exciting moments in any woman's life. It's a special turning point after which your priorities change. Now that a baby is on the way, you have to plan and prepare for the future. Maintaining good health is important, as is your emotional well-being. You'll also have a great number of practical questions: when you will deliver, what foods you should eat or avoid and what is actually happening to you and your baby.

PREGNANT!

Many women "know" when they conceive. This special intuitive feeling is probably due to the very early outpouring of female hormones, initially prolonged high levels of progesterone (which a woman does not experience unless she is pregnant), followed by the production of human chorionic gonadotrophin (hCG) by the fetal tissues as soon as the embryo achieves implantation, about seven days after fertilization.

SUSPECTING THAT YOU ARE PREGNANT

There are certain classic signs that can make you suspect that you are pregnant before seeking confirmation.

Amenorrhoea   Within two weeks of fertilization, a woman may miss a period. Although pregnancy is the most common cause of amenorrhoea, it is not the only one, so a missed period should not be taken as an absolute sign of pregnancy. Several other factors such as jet lag, severe illness, surgery, shock, bereavement or great stress also can cause amenorrhoea. Periods, however, do not always stop in pregnancy: some women have been known to have light periods up to the sixth month, and occasionally throughout their pregnancies.

Frequency of urination   As soon as progesterone levels rise and the embryo starts to secrete hCG, the blood supply to the pelvic area increases, which leads to pelvic congestion. This is then communicated to the bladder, which itself becomes irritable and tries to expel even the smallest quantity of urine. Most women therefore experience the desire to urinate more frequently than usual. This can happen as early as one week after conception.

Tiredness   Fatigue is partly due to very high levels of progesterone, which has a sedative effect. During early pregnancy your metabolism speeds up in order to support your developing embryo and your vital organs, which have to cope with an increased amount of work. This can lead to extreme fatigue, which is sometimes so great that you just have to sleep.

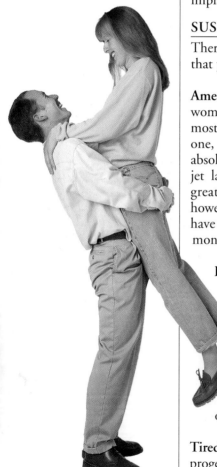

Discovering a new life
Finding out you are pregnant can be one of the most special moments in your life.

Odd tastes and cravings The saliva often reflects the chemical content of the blood and, with rising hormone levels, the taste within your mouth can change, often being described as metallic. This can also make certain foods taste different than they normally do, with some that you may usually enjoy (coffee is a common example) even becoming intolerable. There is no real scientific explanation for cravings, which can occasionally be for very odd things such as coal, but they are thought to be the body's response to deficiency in certain minerals and trace elements. Try to control cravings for inedible substances, as well as for high-calorie junk foods.

Morning sickness Most common in the morning, morning sickness can come on at any time of day especially when you do not eat often enough and your blood sugar drops as a result.

Smell Pregnancy often heightens your sense of smell and you may find that common odours such as cooking smells make you nauseous.

Breast changes Even at the start of pregnancy, breast changes may be quite obvious: your breasts can become quite lumpy and sore to the touch; the nipple area may become tender and sensitive, and will deepen in colour; and veins can become enlarged.

CONFIRMING PREGNANCY

Once you suspect that you are pregnant you should seek confirmation as soon as possible. There are a variety of tests available. Some are more accurate than others.

Blood test This test has to be performed by your doctor and it can accurately detect the fetal hormone hCG (human chorionic gonadotrophin) in the blood as early as two weeks after conception – about the time your next period is due.

Urine test HCG can also be detected by means of a urine test. These are widely available and are over 90 per cent reliable. They can be performed as soon as two weeks after conception, although you will get the most reliable result if you wait four weeks longer (see also p. 10).

TELLING THE WORLD

You will obviously tell your partner, and possibly your immediate family, as soon as you know yourself.

Doctor *Your pregnancy may be confirmed by your doctor, so he or she will obviously know immediately. If not, you should get in contact as soon as you can to discuss birth options and antenatal care.*

Employer *You should tell your employer before you attend your first antenatal clinic (see p. 22), which will probably be at about three months.*

Friends and acquaintances *Many women delay telling friends and acquaintances that they are pregnant until after the first three months. Although this is understandable, it is probably unnecessary once your doctor has confirmed your pregnancy.*

DO YOU HAVE THE CORRECT RESULT?

A number of factors can affect whether your pregnancy test results are accurate.

- *In older women, hormonal changes caused by approaching menopause can give false positives or negatives.*

- *Improperly collected or stored urine can lead to errors.*

- *If the test is performed too early, the concentration of hCG will be too low to detect. It is important to know when your period was due. Irregular or infrequent periods can affect the accuracy of the test.*

- *Antidepressant or fertility drugs can change the results. Contraceptive pills, antibiotics and painkillers should not have any effect.*

- *If the equipment used for the test is too hot, the result may be false. Urine must be at room temperature when tested.*

HOME TESTING

Many women prefer to find out whether they are pregnant in the privacy of their own homes because they can be sure of complete confidentiality. There are a variety of pregnancy testing kits available from chemists; these are simple to use and offer immediate results with an accuracy rate exceeding 90 percent.

How the tests work All the urine tests check for the presence of hCG (human chorionic gonadotrophin), the hormone manufactured by the blastocyst (fertilized egg). Two of the main types, the ring and the colour tests, involve mixing the chemical solution provided with a sample of your urine. The chemicals react according to the amount of hCG in your urine. The reaction is shown by a colour change in the tube or window strip, or coagulation is prevented, thereby causing the appearance of a dark ring in the tube. A third test can be performed by simply placing the absorbent part of the test strip in contact with the urine. From two weeks after conception, hCG may be detected in urine. Most kits advise using the test between one and four days after the first day of your missed period. However, if you do perform the test then, repeat it two weeks later when the hCG is more concentrated and the result will be more reliable. Most kits provide two tests for the purpose of confirmation.

Necessary precautions Collect a sample of urine in a clean, soap-free container first thing in the morning (it will have a higher concentration of hCG). Do not drink any liquids before the test since this will dilute the sample. Follow the kit's instructions very carefully and do not use the test if it has been damaged in any way. If you cannot perform the test immediately, store the specimen in the refrigerator, but only for up to 12 hours.

Unexpected result There is the possibility that a test will show a positive result that becomes negative when repeated and your period may start a few days later. Don't worry. Half of all conceptions do not become established pregnancies because the implanted egg fails to become established in the uterus and there is a natural abortion (possibly because of an abnormality). The test was positive because it was done before the loss of the fertilized egg. To avoid this, do the test around the time of your first missed period. If there is a weak but positive result, repeat the test a few days later with a fresh sample.

EXPECTED ARRIVAL DATE

Once you have confirmed that you are pregnant, your next question is almost certainly, "When will my baby be born?". About 266 days or 38 weeks pass between conception and birth. This is the same as 40 weeks from the start of your last menstrual period (LMP) because ovulation, and therefore conception, is normally two weeks after the start of your last period (see chart, below). You can work out the approximate date of the baby's arrival with calculations using the first day of your last period. The accuracy of this date is dependent on a regular 28-day cycle. If you have a shorter or longer menstrual cycle, your delivery date will probably differ slightly.

YOUR BABY'S ARRIVAL

The EDD (Estimated Delivery Date) is only approximate. You should be flexible about this and not see it as the exact day that you will go into labour. A healthy pregnancy may last between 38 and 42 weeks.

How the chart works
Find the first day of your last period on the chart by looking for the month in bold type, and then look along the line to the actual date. The figure below it is your baby's estimated date of delivery.

YOUR ESTIMATED DATE OF DELIVERY

January	1	2	3	4	5	6	7	8	9	10	11	12	13	14	15	16	17	18	19	20	21	22	23	24	25	26	27	28	29	30	31
Oct/Nov	8	9	10	11	12	13	14	15	16	17	18	19	20	21	22	23	24	25	26	27	28	29	30	31	1	2	3	4	5	6	7
February	1	2	3	4	5	6	7	8	9	10	11	12	13	14	15	16	17	18	19	20	21	22	23	24	25	26	27	28			
Nov/Dec	8	9	10	11	12	13	14	15	16	17	18	19	20	21	22	23	24	25	26	27	28	29	30	1	2	3	4	5			
March	1	2	3	4	5	6	7	8	9	10	11	12	13	14	15	16	17	18	19	20	21	22	23	24	25	26	27	28	29	30	31
Dec/Jan	6	7	8	9	10	11	12	13	14	15	16	17	18	19	20	21	22	23	24	25	26	27	28	29	30	31	1	2	3	4	5
April	1	2	3	4	5	6	7	8	9	10	11	12	13	14	15	16	17	18	19	20	21	22	23	24	25	26	27	28	29	30	
Jan/Feb	6	7	8	9	10	11	12	13	14	15	16	17	18	19	20	21	22	23	24	25	26	27	28	29	30	31	1	2	3	4	
May	1	2	3	4	5	6	7	8	9	10	11	12	13	14	15	16	17	18	19	20	21	22	23	24	25	26	27	28	29	30	31
Feb/Mar	5	6	7	8	9	10	11	12	13	14	15	16	17	18	19	20	21	22	23	24	25	26	27	28	1	2	3	4	5	6	7
June	1	2	3	4	5	6	7	8	9	10	11	12	13	14	15	16	17	18	19	20	21	22	23	24	25	26	27	28	29	30	
Mar/April	8	9	10	11	12	13	14	15	16	17	18	19	20	21	22	23	24	25	26	27	28	29	30	31	1	2	3	4	5	6	
July	1	2	3	4	5	6	7	8	9	10	11	12	13	14	15	16	17	18	19	20	21	22	23	24	25	26	27	28	29	30	31
April/May	7	8	9	10	11	12	13	14	15	16	17	18	19	20	21	22	23	24	25	26	27	28	29	30	1	2	3	4	5	6	7
August	1	2	3	4	5	6	7	8	9	10	11	12	13	14	15	16	17	18	19	20	21	22	23	24	25	26	27	28	29	30	31
May/June	8	9	10	11	12	13	14	15	16	17	18	19	20	21	22	23	24	25	26	27	28	29	30	31	1	2	3	4	5	6	7
September	1	2	3	4	5	6	7	8	9	10	11	12	13	14	15	16	17	18	19	20	21	22	23	24	25	26	27	28	29	30	
June/July	8	9	10	11	12	13	14	15	16	17	18	19	20	21	22	23	24	25	26	27	28	29	30	1	2	3	4	5	6	7	
October	1	2	3	4	5	6	7	8	9	10	11	12	13	14	15	16	17	18	19	20	21	22	23	24	25	26	27	28	29	30	31
July/Aug	8	9	10	11	12	13	14	15	16	17	18	19	20	21	22	23	24	25	26	27	28	29	30	31	1	2	3	4	5	6	7
November	1	2	3	4	5	6	7	8	9	10	11	12	13	14	15	16	17	18	19	20	21	22	23	24	25	26	27	28	29	30	
Aug/Sept	8	9	10	11	12	13	14	15	16	17	18	19	20	21	22	23	24	25	26	27	28	29	30	31	1	2	3	4	5	6	
December	1	2	3	4	5	6	7	8	9	10	11	12	13	14	15	16	17	18	19	20	21	22	23	24	25	26	27	28	29	30	31
Sept/Oct	7	8	9	10	11	12	13	14	15	16	17	18	19	20	21	22	23	24	25	26	27	28	29	30	1	2	3	4	5	6	7

FIRST TRIMESTER

During pregnancy, the trimesters are the major milestones for the mother-to-be. Rather than representing three three-monthly periods, they are periods of uneven length, and are defined by the rate of fetal growth. By convention, the trimesters date from presumed conception (two weeks after your last period), and the first trimester represents the first 12 weeks of your baby's fetal life. The second trimester ends at 28 weeks, and the third trimester encompasses the rest of your pregnancy.

During the first trimester, your body adjusts to pregnancy. At the beginning you won't look pregnant, and you may not feel pregnant either, but the activities of your hormones will soon start to affect you in various ways. Your moods may change capriciously, your libido may decrease or increase, and you may find that your appetite changes and that you prefer blander food.

PHYSICAL CHANGES

Your pregnant body has to work very hard to accommodate the developing embryo and the placenta. Pregnancy induces a higher metabolic rate – between ten percent and 25 percent higher than normal – which means that the body accelerates all of its functions. Your heart's blood output rises steeply, almost to the maximum level that will be maintained throughout the rest of the pregnancy. Your heartbeat rate rises too, and will continue to do so until the middle of the second trimester. Your breathing becomes more rapid as you now send more oxygen to the fetus and exhale more carbon dioxide.

Owing to the action of oestrogen and progesterone, your breasts quickly become larger and heavier, and are usually tender to the touch from very early on. Fatty deposits are increased and new milk ducts grow. The areola around the nipple becomes darker and develops little nodules called Montgomery's tubercles. As the blood supply to the breasts increases, you will notice a network of bluish lines appearing underneath the skin.

Your uterus enlarges even in early pregnancy, but it cannot be felt through the abdominal wall until the end of the first trimester, when it begins to rise above the pelvic brim. Your uterus will increasingly press upon your bladder as it enlarges, so you will need to urinate

Early days
In the first trimester, you may experience nausea and fatigue but the visible changes to your body will be slight and you will not need to buy new clothes yet.

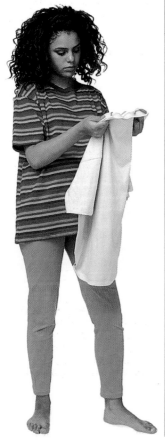

more often. In addition, the muscle fibres of your uterus begin to thicken until it becomes very solid. However, you probably won't notice any increase in your waistline until the end of this trimester.

TAKING CARE OF YOURSELF

You need more carbohydrates and protein to provide nutrients for your growing baby, so it is imperative that you eat healthily from the beginning of your pregnancy (see p. 18). You will need more fluids, so try to drink at least eight glasses of water a day. Make sure, too, that you are getting plenty of rest. Drugs, alcohol, smoking, caffeine and junk food should be avoided in pregnancy.

Clothes While there is probably no need to invest in maternity clothes just yet, there's nothing worse than having to put up with tight clothes and being uncomfortable, so make sure that you stay one step ahead of your increasing size. However, you are likely to need a larger support bra early on, and it should be a properly fitted maternity bra.

YOUR ANTENATAL CARE

Your doctor may be the one who confirms your pregnancy, or you may make an appointment with the antenatal clinic as soon as you have a positive test result. If this is the case, you may not be seen until your next trimester. At the first visit, you will be asked questions about yourself, your partner and both of your families' medical histories, and you will have a thorough physical examination, which will include urine and blood tests.

Making plans

Your doctor will be able to advise you about the childbirth options available in your area, and may offer antenatal care, whether complete or shared with your hospital. You will need to start thinking about the type of delivery you want and where you are most likely to get it. Books like this one can help you determine your choices in childbirth as well as provide in-depth information.

YOUR PREGNANCY

Finding out that you are pregnant, especially for the first time, is extremely exciting, and you will undoubtedly long for the physical signs that will confirm the pregnancy test.

- *Your breasts will grow larger, heavier and more sensitive.*

- *The pigmentation of your nipples and freckles will darken.*

- *You may feel very tired.*

- *You will probably experience nausea, especially first thing in the morning.*

- *You will need to urinate frequently.*

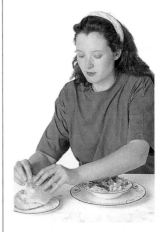

Your appetite in pregnancy
Your tastes in food will change. You may experience strange tastes in the mouth, unusual food cravings or entirely go off foods that you normally like.

SECOND TRIMESTER

Now is the time when pregnancy is well established and many of the minor complaints associated with early pregnancy have disappeared. It is, however, the time when certain tests may need to be done. Amniocentesis (see p. 56), for example, will be offered to women over 35, those with a family history of congenital abnormalities, and those who have suffered repeated miscarriages.

PHYSICAL CHANGES

You may notice that your nipples begin to secrete colostrum, which is the "pre-milk" that you first feed your baby with. Your waistline will disappear and you will now "look" pregnant. Your gums may become slightly spongy, probably owing to the action of pregnancy hormones. However, there is no evidence for increased dental decay during pregnancy and absolutely no evidence to suggest that there is any truth in the saying "a tooth lost for every child".

Digestion The entire musculature of your intestinal tract is relaxed and this is the cause of many of the minor discomforts in pregnancy. Oesophageal reflux may cause heartburn because of the relaxation of the sphincter at the top of the stomach. Gastric emptying is less efficient and therefore the food remains for longer in the stomach. The relaxed intestinal muscle also leads to fewer bowel movements and although this permits more complete absorption of foods, it can also often lead to constipation during pregnancy.

Your increasing size Generally speaking, once your uterus has expanded above your pelvis, your waistline will begin to disappear and you will need to wear larger and looser clothing. Yet the second trimester is a classic time for women to be told that they look small for their expected delivery dates. If this happens to you, don't worry. How big you look will depend on many factors including your height and build; whether this is your first pregnancy or not – because the uterine muscle tends to get stretched after the first child; and the size of your baby. If your doctor is satisfied with the progress of pregnancy, you should be too.

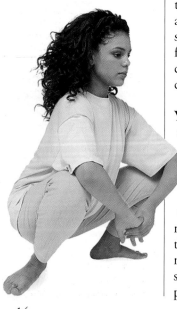

Take it slow and easy
Without overdoing it, enjoy the burst of glowing health and energy you should feel during the second trimester. Regular exercises and relaxation are beneficial during this time.

TAKING CARE OF YOURSELF

This is the trimester in which you will gain the most weight overall (approximately 6kg/12lb) and it is essential that you continue to eat well (see p. 18). Your posture may change as the muscles of the abdominal wall become stretched in order to accommodate your enlarging uterus. Your centre of gravity alters because you are carrying an increasing amount of weight in front. Leaning backwards to try to counter this may result in backache.

Backache Apart from bad posture (see above), backache is caused by the increased blood flow to your pelvis, and the rise in hormones. These cause some softening and relaxation of the ligaments of the sacroiliac joints (the sacrum), which attach your pelvic bones to your spine at the back. In addition, the ligaments and the cartilage at the front of your pelvis loosen and these joints become more mobile.

To help prevent backache, sit with your back straight and don't slouch, don't wear high-heeled shoes, and preferably sit on a hard chair or the floor. Always keep your back straight if you have to lift anything, bend from the knees and lift from a crouching position.

YOUR ANTENATAL CARE

Regular checks of your urine, weight and blood pressure may be augmented by testing for chromosomal defects. During the fourth month you may have a routine ultrasound scan, and you will have the excitement of seeing your baby for the first time. You will be able to hear the incredibly fast heartbeat and may see your baby moving.

PREPARING FOR BABY

Towards the end of this trimester, when you are feeling well and full of energy, is the ideal time to prepare your baby's room and shop for the layette and baby equipment. You can also begin to assemble (and have ready to pack in your hospital bag) the items you will need during labour.

YOUR PREGNANCY

During the second trimester you will begin to feel comfortable with being pregnant. You will enjoy the sensation of your baby moving within you and will feel energetic and full of life.

- *Your libido will return or increase.*

- *Your abdomen will become rounded. You will lose your waistline and "look" pregnant.*

- *Pigmentation will continue to increase and you may notice a darker line developing down the centre of your abdomen – the linea nigra.*

- *You may suffer from indigestion and rib pain.*

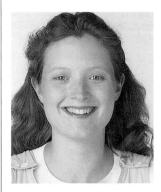

Hormonal effects
As the placenta takes over the production of pregnancy hormones, your hormone levels should begin to balance out. This means that you will feel more serene and positive than you did in the first trimester. Your appearance will also benefit, with thicker and shinier hair and clear and glowing skin.

THIRD TRIMESTER

You will probably feel anxious about labour and wish you could have the baby now. This doesn't mean that there is anything wrong with your baby. The sense of urgency is due to metabolic changes in the brain. Subtle shifts have gone on in each trimester, bringing about the fatigue of the first, the elation and vigour of the second, and now the anxiety and impatience of the third.

PHYSICAL CHANGES

Your size is now increasing rapidly and you are bound to feel tired. You may find that you are not sleeping at night as well as usual and this will mean you will need more daytime rest. As your ligaments stretch and give way, you may find walking about increasingly uncomfortable. Once your baby has settled into your pelvis (called engagement), you will find that your discomfort and breathlessness will diminish because the pressure on your diaphragm has been relieved.

Breathing As the baby grows bigger in the abdomen, there is reduced space for the diaphragm so pregnant women breathe more deeply and take more air in with each breath; this allows for better mixing of gases and more efficient consumption of oxygen. This has the effect of increasing the amount of air per breath from 500 mililitres to 700 mililitres (from 17.5 to 24.5 fluid ounces), an increase of over 40 percent. It also means that more carbon dioxide than normal is exhaled per breath. The low level of carbon dioxide in the blood makes you feel you are short of breath and this may be troublesome during this trimester. Relief should come when your baby engages in your pelvis and the diaphragm can once again work efficiently; your breathing rate will settle back to normal. Meanwhile, sit in a slightly propped-up position and avoid overdoing things.

CARING FOR YOURSELF

As the third trimester continues, the extra weight you are carrying can result in further backache and cause you to feel continually tired. Sleep can become a problem as you get bigger, since very few positions in bed seem to be comfortable. Don't be

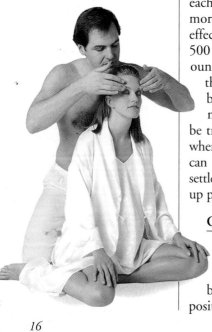

Help with relaxation
If you are having trouble getting to sleep, you may find that a loving massage can help you relax.

tempted to take sleeping pills because they will make the baby sleepy too. Take your time with everything during the last month, and make sure that you get adequate rest; catnap whenever you can and set aside periods when you can relax, even if you don't sleep. As your desire for making love may diminish or be frustrated by your increasing size, you may find that massage can enable you to relax and unwind, particularly if your partner can make it sensual. Continue to eat lots of fresh fruit and vegetables and drink at least eight glasses of fluid per day because you'll probably urinate more often. This will also help relieve constipation.

YOUR ANTENATAL CARE

There are many tests that your doctor may use to judge the baby's health or well-being, such as ultrasound, fetal heart rate monitoring and hormonal measurements, and your doctor will discuss at each stage what is being done and why. Unlike the special tests in the second trimester – amniocentesis, chorionic villus sampling and cordocentesis (see pp. 56–7 & 58–9) – none of the tests at this time is invasive of the uterus. Urine and blood pressure testing will be done frequently, as will checks for possible swelling of your feet and hands. From the 36th week until the onset of labour, you will be seen at more frequent intervals.

PREPARING FOR BABY

Towards the end of this trimester you should have completed your baby's layette, sorted out the baby's room, and purchased the essential equipment. Some women stop working by the seventh month, and if you have done so, you will be able to take life at your own pace. Labour may be increasingly on your mind, and some women do find themselves worrying almost obsessively about it. Although no-one can predict exactly what will happen during your labour, because every experience is unique, be reassured that the majority of births are normal and successful.

YOUR PREGNANCY

Practical matters such as attending childbirth classes and preparing your baby's clothes and room will vie with daydreaming about the new arrival.

• *You will probably get tired easily and you may find it hard to sleep at night.*

• *You will become increasingly aware of Braxton Hicks' contractions as your uterus practises for labour.*

• *You will have visited the hospital and become familiar with it and the staff. If you are having a home birth, you will have ready all the items you will need.*

You may be concerned about whether you can tell if you are in labour. Even for an experienced midwife or doctor, it is difficult to know when you are in real labour. The classic signs are regular and long contractions and the appearance of the "show" or your waters breaking.

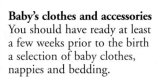

Baby's clothes and accessories
You should have ready at least a few weeks prior to the birth a selection of baby clothes, nappies and bedding.

EATING FOR YOURSELF

Your body will never work harder than it does during pregnancy and childbirth. To cope with the increased demands, maintain your strength and enjoy your pregnancy, you must eat well.

• *Increase your intake by 500 calories per day.*

• *Start to eat 5–6 small meals a day instead of 2–3 big ones.*

• *Make certain you get enough protein and carbohydrates; the former supplies essential nutrients for your developing baby, the latter meets your energy needs.*

• *Eat foods that contain vitamins, such as vitamin C, and minerals, particularly iron (see below).*

EATING FOR YOUR BABY

During pregnancy, you are your baby's only source of nourishment. Every calorie, vitamin or gram of protein that your baby needs must be eaten by you. Only you can make sure that the best quality food reaches her.

Your baby needs extra protein and iron to develop well. You will fulfil all of your baby's requirements if you eat lots of fruit, green leafy vegetables, beans, peas, wholemeal cereals and pasta, fish, fowl and low-fat dairy products. Try to include iron-rich foods such as red meat, eggs, apricots, raisins and prunes.

DIET IN PREGNANCY

Pregnant women, like most people, rarely have the time or inclination to sit around measuring out ounces of this and portions of that and trying to remember the calorific value of everything. In fact, there's no need to do that as long as you follow some basic guidelines about healthy eating in pregnancy. One important rule is that the nearer food is to its natural state, the more nutritious it is. So fresh food is best, frozen is next best, and you should always make tinned foods your last choice. In many ways, good nutrition is just common sense.

EATING FOR TWO?

As your pregnancy progresses your appetite will increase; this is nature's way of making certain you eat enough for you and your baby. Your energy requirements will increase only by 15 percent, or 500 calories per day, far less than if you ate twice your normal amount of food. The saying "eating for two", therefore, is dangerous to follow because you'll end up putting on weight, which is extremely difficult to lose afterwards. Everything you eat should be good for you and your baby. More problems develop if you eat too little rather than too much – pregnancy is not the time for dieting. It is best to balance your food intake over a 24- to 48-hour period rather than at each meal.

DAILY REQUIREMENTS

To give you and your baby the best possible diet, try to eat the following portions each day. You should vary the food you choose:

• Proteins (meat, fish, eggs, cheese) – 3 servings
• Calcium-rich foods (cheese, milk, tinned sardines with bones) – 4 servings during pregnancy, 5 while breast-feeding
• Vitamin C foods (green leafy and yellow vegetables and fruits) – 3 servings
• Other fruit and vegetables – 1 or 2 servings
• Whole grains and complex carbohydrates (brown rice, wholemeal bread or pasta) – 4 or 5 servings
• Iron-rich food (eggs, red meat, cereals) – 2 servings
• Fluids – drink at least 8 glasses of water a day

ESSENTIAL NUTRITION

Carbohydrates Carbohydrates are the essential fuel that gives you energy. Most of your calories should come from carbohydrates, but rather than sugar-based carbohydrates, you should eat mostly complex carbohydrates in the form of wholemeal bread, porridge, brown rice, potatoes, peas, beans and lentils because these provide long-lasting energy and fibre. Avoid processed carbohydrates where possible. However, simple carbohydrates are absorbed by the system in minutes, so the sugars from fructose (fruit), lactose (milk) and dextrose (honey) are good for a quick energy boost and can help to relieve morning sickness.

Protein Protein is the building block to enable all your baby's tissues – bone, muscle, cartilage and blood to grow, so you should eat at least 100g (4oz) of protein a day if you can. You may not necessarily eat red meat very often (or at all) but in pregnancy it is important because red meat is the most concentrated source of iron (see p. 20). For vegetarians, milk (skimmed), yoghurt, cheese and eggs are excellent sources of protein; so is the vegetable protein in seeds, nuts, peanut butter (though calorific), as well as in peas, beans and lentils. Most bread is protein-enriched. Eat as much fish as you can – it's easily digested pure protein, rich in minerals and vitamins – oily fish also contain essential fatty acids.

Vitamins All the vitamins are important for maintaining general good health but some vitamins such as B and C cannot be stored by the body and a daily intake is required. The B vitamins are supplied in some vegetables and fruit and are also found in meat, fish, dairy products, grains and nuts. Vitamin C is provided by fresh fruit and vegetables. Vitamin D is found in fish oils and can be manufactured by the body if it is triggered by the action of light on the skin; most people in the UK require about 40 minutes of sunlight per day to produce adequate amounts. Folic acid is important in the prevention of spina bifida and supplements should be taken for three months before you get pregnant and during the first trimester. Avoid liver or liver pâtés because they are high in vitamin A which can cause problems in pregnancy.

YOUR WEIGHT GAIN

Doctors recommend that a woman of average weight, experiencing an average pregnancy, ought to gain an average of 10–13kg (22–28lb) in the total 40 weeks' gestation. This allows about 3–4kg (6–8lb) for the baby and about 7–9kg (15–20lb) for the baby's support system (comprising placenta, amniotic fluid, increased blood, fluid, fat and breast tissue).

- *During the first trimester you will probably gain very little, about 1–2kg (2–4lb), if nausea hasn't been a problem. Of this, only 48g (1.7oz) will be your baby. The rest is made up of the baby's support system.*

- *During the second trimester, you will probably gain approximately 6kg (12lb). Of this, only 1kg (2lb) will actually be your baby. The rest is made up of the baby's support system.*

- *During the third trimester you will probably gain about 5kg (10lb). Of this, approximately 3–4kg (6–8lb) will be accounted for by your baby. The rest is made up of the baby's support system.*

A steady gain like this means that your body can adapt more easily to your increasing size; if you are eating regularly, your baby has a continuous flow of nourishment.

PREPARING FOOD

Try to develop some good cooking habits that will promote a healthy eating style.

- *Trim the fat from meat before cooking.*

- *Skim the fat off the surface of casseroles and soups.*

- *Bake, steam, mircrowave or grill rather than fry.*

- *Stir-fry in a teaspoon of olive oil, or simmer with a stock cube dissolved in a cup of water.*

- *Use non-stick pans and the minimum of fat when cooking.*

- *Add dried skimmed milk to milky drinks for extra calcium.*

- *Always choose low-fat (not full-fat) dairy products.*

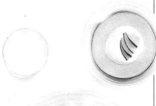

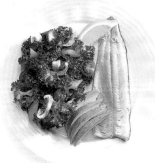

A balanced meal
Salmon trout and salad, with melon, yoghurt and nectarine to follow, and a glass of milk make a nutritious meal.

Minerals These are essential for your body to function efficiently. As soon as you conceive, calcium is needed to build your baby's skeleton and teeth. Keep your calcium intake high by eating broccoli, dried milk and tinned salmon with the bones. Green leafy vegetables and dairy products also contain calcium. Remember that vitamin D is needed to promote calcium absorption.

Iron This is vital, not just for your baby but for your own needs too. Your baby uses iron so fast that he is, so to speak, in a constant iron-deficient state. If you are iron-deficient when you become pregnant, or become so later on, your doctor will prescribe iron tablets or injections to prevent you from developing anaemia. Eat plenty of foods that are rich in iron, such as red meat, eggs, apricots, raisins and prunes, but avoid liver.

VEGETARIAN DIETS

If you do not eat meat, you need to ensure you get enough protein, vitamins and iron to meet your own and your baby's needs from other sources. Animal products also provide calcium, vitamins B^6, B^{12} and D, which are essential for health; vitamin B^{12} supplements may be necessary if you eat no animal products.

WHAT TO AVOID

Certain common precautions should be taken because we now know that some foods are contaminated with enough numbers of bacteria to cause illness, and may even cause miscarriage or birth defects.

Listeria is a rare bacterium found in soft cheeses, unpasteurized milk, ready-made coleslaw, cooked chilled foods, pâtés and improperly cooked meat. Bacteria are normally destroyed at pasteurizing temperatures, but if food is infected and refrigerated, the bacteria may continue to multiply. Also, wash your hands after any direct contact with infected animals, such as sheep.

Salmonella is a bacterium found in eggs and chicken that causes fever, abdominal pain and severe diarrhoea. It is killed by thorough cooking.

Toxoplasmosis is caused by a parasite found in cat and dog faeces and also in raw meat. It can cause birth defects. Always wash your hands after handling a pet or its litter tray and wear gloves when gardening.

ROUTINE
EARLY CARE

Excellent antenatal care should be rewarded with healthy

mothers and babies. Routine tests will usually spot any

problems as soon as they arise, while special tests are

available for mothers and babies with particular needs.

Furthermore, a relaxed and informed mother is more likely

to have a positive labour and delivery. The antenatal clinic

also provides opportunities to ask questions and to meet

other women going through the same experience as

yourself. It is a good idea to take the time now to discuss

with your hospital or midwife your options about how

your labour and delivery will be handled.

There are many different approaches to birth, so ask your main carer (whether it is your obstetrician or midwife) the following questions to find out exactly what you can expect from him or her.

• *What are your views on inducing labour?*

• *Under what circumstances would you consider it necessary to rupture the membranes?*

• *Do you believe electronic fetal monitoring is a valuable aid in every birth?*

• *Would you be concerned if labour was slower than normal?*

• *What are your views on moving about, the use of water or a birth pool, and breathing techniques to help relieve pain? What drugs do you normally give to control pain?*

• *Would you be concerned if the lights were dimmed during labour?*

• *How often do you perform episiotomies?*

• *Are you happy for me to stand or squat to deliver my baby?*

• *Under what conditions would you consider a Caesarean section to be necessary?*

• *Will we be able to have some time alone with our baby immediately after his birth?*

YOUR PROFESSIONAL CARERS

There are a number of options open to you regarding who attends your labour – it does not have to be a straight choice between hospital expertise or a home midwife. Wherever you decide to have your baby, the system can usually be tailored to suit your individual needs. Of course, the professional attendant is not the only one you should think about. Many women are supported by their partners or a friend during childbirth, and most hospitals now welcome this.

YOUR OWN GP

Your general practitioner will probably be the first professional person that you see. You need to establish his or her views on birth – especially if you are interested in having a home birth. A few doctors are happy to attend a home delivery of a normal pregnancy, many are not so willing, some fall somewhere in between – preferring you to have had at least one straightforward delivery in hospital first. Many doctors provide antenatal care if you are having the baby in the hospital to which they have referred you. Occasionally you may be able to attend your doctor's clinic even if you are booked into another hospital – try to explore all of the options.

GP units Some areas still have separate small (cottage) hospitals staffed by midwives and local general practitioners, while some hospitals have GP units as part of their care. The main advantages of these are that you are guaranteed continuation of care, that you know the people who will be assisting you, and that you can successfully combine medical back-up with the advantages of home.

CONSULTANTS AND OBSTETRICIANS

An obstetrician is a consultant who specializes in medical problems to do with pregnancy and childbirth. When you book into a hospital you will be assigned to an obstetrician. You can ask to be referred to a particular obstetrician, although that consultant is not obliged to take you. Obstetricians tend to be male, although the number of female obstetricians is rising – if you feel strongly that you want a woman obstetrician, check with your hospital. If they have one, you should make this preference clear on your birth plan. There is, however, no guarantee that the obstetrician of your choice will be on duty when you go into labour.

You will be unlikely to see your consultant unless you have problems in your pregnancy. Most routine care is provided by junior doctors working alongside midwives in the obstetrics team.

MIDWIVES

The modern, professional midwife is a specialist in childbirth, qualified to take responsibility for you before, during, and after the birth. She is able to support and understand you during labour and delivery, and knows when to call for obstetric advice and assistance. Unlike the obstetrician, her focus is on the normal not the abnormal. Midwives working outside hospitals tend to be more flexible than hospital carers.

Domino and team midwives Midwives who are working under the "domino" (DOMiciliary IN and Out) scheme or who are part of the team midwife scheme, provide a more personal service. One midwife or a team of midwives is allocated to you; a midwife will come to your house for antenatal care and when labour starts, go with you to the hospital to deliver your baby; your GP and hospital staff are only rarely involved. If all goes well, you are usually discharged from hospital within a few hours of the birth into her care.

Independent midwives These midwives provide continuous care in a variety of situations. They will deliver you wherever you choose, whether at home or in hospital and undertake to be with you throughout the labour and delivery (see also column, right).

Hospital midwives In a few hospitals midwives are used as subordinate members of teams headed by obstetricians. They may only be responsible for menial tasks such as weighing you and keeping records. However, in most hospitals, there are now midwives who will deliver you with the minimum of obstetric intervention.

INDEPENDENT MIDWIVES

Because your midwife will be your primary caregiver you will need to get to know her. You may like to ask her the following questions:

- *What training and experience has she had?*

- *Does she work alone, or with other midwives? Will you be able to meet them?*

- *What are her considerations in managing labour?*

- *What is her back-up system? Does she work closely with any doctors?*

- *What equipment, drugs and resuscitation equipment for the baby does she carry?*

- *What antenatal care does she provide? Are there home visits?*

- *Under what conditions would she transfer you to hospital?*

YOUR FIRST VISIT

On your first visit to the antenatal clinic, you will be asked questions about:

- *Your personal details and circumstances.*

- *Childhood illnesses or serious illnesses you have had.*

- *Any illnesses that run in your family, or in your partner's family.*

- *If there are twins in your family.*

- *Your menstrual history and the date of your last menstrual period.*

- *Your pregnancy symptoms, and your general health.*

- *Details of previous births, pregnancies, or problems in conceiving.*

- *If you take any prescription medicine or have any allergies.*

Discussing your pregnancy
Don't be afraid to ask questions about what is said to you at the clinic.

ANTENATAL CARE

Consultations, check-ups and tests are carried out throughout your pregnancy to ensure a healthy pregnancy. Although most pregnancies proceed normally, these visits and investigations are vital to monitor your progress and spot problems before any harm is done.

THE ANTENATAL CLINIC

You will attend the antenatal clinic at either the hospital where you will have your baby or at your doctor's surgery. Most women attend once a month up until week 32, then every two weeks up to 36 weeks, and then once a week for the last month. You will need to attend more frequently if any complications develop, you're expecting more than one baby, you have a pre-existing medical condition, or if you are at risk of complications.

Attending an antenatal clinic in a large hospital often seems intimidating and frustrating: there are a large number of staff coming and going, and you may be kept waiting for some time. Many women describe it as a cattle market. Negative feelings can be made much worse by the discontinuity of care – it's quite possible to see different nurses and doctors at every visit. Much of this can be avoided if you opt for a GP unit, shared care or the "domino" system (see p. 23) where you mainly see your doctor or your midwife for check-ups with occasional visits to the hospital clinic.

Try to make the best of your time at the antenatal clinic by taking along something to read or to do, and some food just in case the food trolley doesn't come by while you are there. Take a friend or your partner with you for company and support. If you already have children, arrange for them to be looked after if at all possible.

TALKING TO YOUR CARERS

Antenatal clinic visits may not offer sufficient time for mothers to talk to their carers. However, finding out what alternatives are open to you and discussing your preferences, as well as being reassured about any worries and fears you may have, is very important. So be prepared to speak up for yourself and insist on extra time to discuss things. If you have strong preferences but worry that you won't be able to stand up for yourself, take along your partner for moral support. It will probably help if you make a list of issues beforehand.

YOUR FILE

At your first antenatal visit all the details of your past medical and obstetric (if any) history, including your menstrual history, will be noted in your file or booklet.

This file goes with you wherever you go and the contents can be transferred from one set of case notes to another so that your carers have important information about you available and continuity of care is assured. Remember that you must take it with you to the hospital when you go into labour.

The details may initially be difficult to understand since many of the medical terms are abbreviated. Compare the abbreviations on your file or booklet with those that are explained below. If it still does not seem to make much sense, don't hesitate to ask your midwife or doctor.

MEDICAL TERMS AND ABBREVIATIONS

NAD or nil or a tick No abnormality detected.
Alb Albumin in urine (a name for one of the proteins found in the urine sample).
BP Blood pressure.
FH Fetal heart.
FHH/NH Fetal heart heard or not heard.
FMF Fetal movements felt.
Ceph. Cephalic, baby is head down.
Vx Vertex, baby is head down.
Br Breech, baby is bottom down.
Long L Longitudinal lie, the baby is lying parallel to your spine in the uterus.
RSA Right sacrum anterior – the most common breech presentation.
LMP Last menstrual period.
EDD/EDC Estimated date of delivery/confinement.
Hb Haemoglobin levels to check for anaemia.
Eng/E Engaged: the baby's head has dropped down into the pelvis.
NE Not engaged.

Fe Iron has been prescribed.
TCA To come again.
Height of fundus The height of the top of the uterus. The baby pushes this up as it grows and often the height is used to estimate the length of the pregnancy. Some clinics measure the height of the fundus with a tape measure in centimetres.
Relation of PP to brim This is the brim of your pelvis. The presenting part (PP) of the baby to the brim in the later stages of your pregnancy will be the part to be born first.
PET Pre-eclamptic toxaemia.
Oed Oedema.
AFP Alpha-fetoprotein.
CS Caesarean section.
H/T Hypertension (high blood pressure).
MSU Midstream urine sample.
Primigravida This is your first pregnancy.
Multigravida You have had more than one pregnancy.
VE Vaginal examination.

THE LIE OF YOUR BABY

Certain abbreviations describe how the baby is lying, and refer to where the back of the baby's head (occiput) is in relation to your body – on the right or left, to the front (anterior) or back (posterior). ROA, for example, means the back of his head is to the front on your right.

The baby's presentation will affect your labour: the posterior position may slow it down.

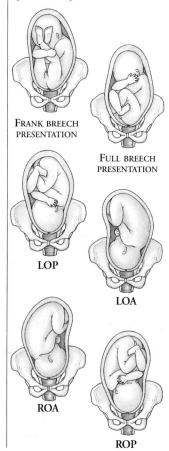

FRANK BREECH PRESENTATION

FULL BREECH PRESENTATION

LOP

LOA

ROA

ROP

BABY'S HEAD SIZE AND YOUR PELVIS

The shape and size of your pelvis is important because of the risk of disproportion, which could become apparent during labour and may delay the baby's delivery.

Disproportion means that your pelvis is too small for your baby's head to pass through it easily, or your baby's head is too large. To avoid delays in delivering your baby, it is important for your doctor or midwife to make an assessment of the size of your pelvic outlet. Your height and shoe size are good guides; short women who have small feet also tend to have small pelvises.

If difficulties are suspected, your baby's head size will be determined by using ultrasound (see p. 32). Severe disproportion will mean delivering the baby by Caesarean section.

Recording your weight
Details of your weight and height are recorded as part of your personal history. You will also be asked about smoking, drinking and street drugs.

ANTENATAL TESTS

Every pregnant woman has certain routine tests to keep a check on her health and the development of her baby; they may be performed at every visit, or at different times during her pregnancy. Some are performed only once. If the tests indicate that there is, or that there may be, a problem, you will be monitored closely and prompt action will be taken if necessary.

HEIGHT AND SHOE SIZE

Your height and shoe size will be noted at your first visit. If you are petite with small feet, you may have a small pelvis, which may need to be assessed. However, the chances are that your baby will be tailored to your physical build and labour will be straightforward.

WEIGHT

This is noted at every visit and gives an indication of the growth of the fetus. You should try to wear the same sort of clothing each time, so that your weight does not fluctuate unnecessarily. In the first trimester a loss of weight usually reflects nausea and vomiting due to morning sickness and is usually nothing to worry about. Sudden weight gain may reflect fluid retention and indicate pre-eclampsia.

In the past, maternal weight gain was taken as a reliable indicator of the growth of the baby. Research now indicates, however, that maternal weight gain should not be relied upon on its own, but viewed in conjunction with external and internal examinations, blood and urine tests, blood pressure and ultrasound scans.

LEGS AND HANDS

At every visit your legs will be checked for varicose veins, and your ankles and hands will be examined for excessive swelling and puffiness (oedema). A little swelling in the final weeks of pregnancy is normal, particularly in the evening and during hot weather. Excessive or sudden swelling does, however, need investigation.

BREASTS

Your breasts will be examined, and the condition of your nipples will be noted. A very few women have dimpled, or inverted, nipples, and these may have to be corrected by wearing a breastshield inside your bra.

URINE

At your first visit and every subsequent visit, a sample of midstream urine (obtained by passing the first few drops into the toilet bowl and collecting a sample of the midstream urine in a sterile container) will be taken to test for the presence of protein, which is a sign of urinary infection; for sugar, to check that you are not developing diabetes; and for ketones, which are the classic sign that diabetes is established and needs urgent treatment. Urine testing in pregnancy can also unmask underlying diabetes. Diabetes may disappear completely after this pregnancy but return in future pregnancies. A trace of protein in your urine in late pregnancy is a strong indication of pre-eclampsia. This will be treated promptly because of the associated potential for miscarriage, a small-for-dates baby and premature delivery.

BLOOD TESTS

At your first visit, a routine blood sample will be taken, usually from a vein in your arm, to find out your basic blood group (O, A, B, AB), and your Rhesus (Rh) blood group (positive or negative), in case a blood transfusion becomes necessary. If you are Rh negative, you will be tested for Rhesus incompatibility (see p. 62). Your haemoglobin level is also ascertained. This is a measure of the oxygen-carrying power of your red blood cells. The normal level is between 12 and 14 grams; if it falls below 10 grams, treatment for anaemia is given. Iron and folic acid raise the oxygen-carrying power of your blood, and prevent anaemia, so make sure you eat iron-rich foods and take folic acid supplements as directed by your doctor.

Further routine and special blood tests may be carried out (see p. 30).

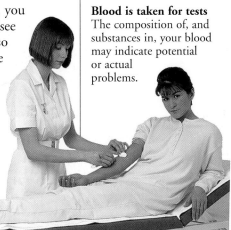

Blood is taken for tests
The composition of, and substances in, your blood may indicate potential or actual problems.

EXTERNAL EXAMINATION

At every visit your abdomen will be palpated (felt) to determine the size of your growing baby. This gives a good idea of whether your baby is approximately the right size for your dates and so is growing well. A series of measurements is taken over the course of your pregnancy that gives a very accurate picture of your baby's rate of progress. The measurement is taken of the distance between your pelvic bone and the top of your uterus (fundus), which normally enlarges into your abdomen at 12 weeks and continues until just prior to term. The amount of amniotic fluid, as well as your individual size and weight, can have an effect on the size of your baby, so after 26–28 weeks the doctor or midwife will also feel for your baby's "poles" (head and rump). This enables them to judge the lie of your baby (see p. 25).

INTERNAL EXAMINATION

By no means will everyone have an internal examination at their first antenatal visit, but if an internal examination is carried out, the doctor or midwife will be able to confirm the pregnancy dates, check your cervix, and, if necessary, assess your pelvic size.

If an internal examination is to be performed, you will be asked to lie down and raise your knees. The doctor or midwife will insert two gloved fingers of one hand into your vagina, and press your abdomen with the other hand to check the size of your uterus to establish whether it is the right size for your dates. If at any time during your pregnancy the baby does not seem to be growing as expected, you will usually have an ultrasound

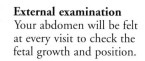

External examination
Your abdomen will be felt at every visit to check the fetal growth and position.

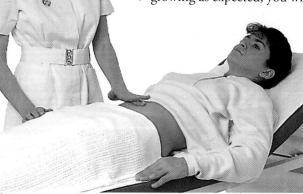

to check this (see p. 32). Your cervix will be examined to see if it's tightly closed, and a cervical smear may be carried out. This is usually a painless scraping of a few cells, which are then sent away to test for abnormal or pre-cancerous cells. As long as you relax, an internal examination is usually only slightly uncomfortable. It will not harm your baby.

Some doctors and midwives will perform another internal examination on certain first-time mothers in order to check their pelvic dimensions. Further internal examinations will be carried out once labour has started.

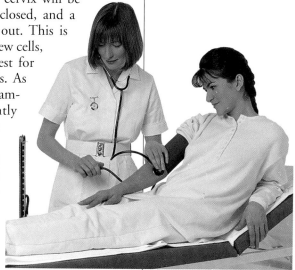

BLOOD PRESSURE

This reading is taken at every visit, and measures the pressure at which your heart is pumping blood through your body. The reading is made up of two figures: the upper one is the systolic pressure – when the heart contracts it pushes out blood and "beats"; this is measured when the arm band is tight. As the pressure is released, the lower, or diastolic, reading is taken; this is the resting pressure between beats.

The statistically average reading in pregnancy is 120 over 70. Blood pressure varies, however, according to your age, and there is a range of blood pressures that is considered normal for each age group. A higher reading than normal may indicate a risk of pre-eclampsia and bed rest in hospital may be advised. Regular antenatal checks ensure that any changes are quickly noted.

Blood pressure
Your blood pressure is taken at every visit and it is a significant measure of how your body is coping with the pregnancy.

FETAL HEARTBEAT

Your baby's heartbeat will be monitored at every visit from week 14. The doctor or midwife may use a sonicaid to listen. This small portable instrument uses ultrasound waves and is placed on your stomach. It magnifies the sound of your baby's heartbeart so that both the midwife and you can listen to it. The baby's heartbeat is almost twice as fast as your own.

ROUTINE BLOOD TESTS

At your first antenatal visit you will have routine blood tests to establish your blood group, your haemoglobin levels and to see whether certain conditions are present. If problems are detected, you will have further, more specific, blood tests.

Blood group and Rhesus (Rh) status Your doctor needs to know which blood group you belong to (A, B, O, AB) in the event of you needing a blood transfusion during the pregnancy or labour. Your Rhesus status is either negative or positive, so that you may be A negative or O positive and so on. If you are Rhesus negative, a further test will be performed to check for the presence of antibodies; tests are repeated at intervals during your pregnancy (see p. 62); your partner will also have to give blood for testing.

Haemoglobin levels The red cells in the blood contain iron and carry oxygen; if the test shows that the number of red cells is low, or that they are short of iron, you will be advised to eat iron-rich foods or take iron tablets.

Rubella (German measles) This blood test shows whether you are have developed immunity to the disease. If not, you could contract rubella in early pregnancy; this could cause heart defects, blindness and deafness in the baby.

Syphilis This sexually transmitted disease is rare these days because it is now so easily cured. If you have the disease and it is not treated during pregnancy, it could cause serious developmental or congenital problems.

Hepatitis B This liver disease is caused by a virus. It can be passed to the baby and cause serious liver damage.

SPECIAL BLOOD TESTS

Triple or Bart's test (for Down's syndrome) It depends on the hospital's policy but this test is usually offered to women with a higher risk of having a Down's baby, for example, those over the age of 35 (see p.60). It shows the level of three substances in the mother's bloodstream; alpha-fetoprotein (AFP) (see column, right), oestriol, and human chorionic gonadotrophin (hCG).

However, because this test screens only, if it is positive it merely means that you have an increased *risk* of a Down's baby. To diagnose this or rule it out, you need an invasive test such as an amniocentesis (see p. 56).

Glucose tolerance test (for diabetes) This test is necessary if you have high blood sugar, sugar in the urine, a large baby, or had diabetes in a previous pregnancy.

The test involves having a sugary drink, after which four samples of blood are taken over the next two hours. If your blood sugar level remains high, it may indicate the presence of diabetes.

Treatment includes strict control of your diet, possibly also with insulin injections, and extra antenatal check-ups. You may also be required to have more than the average two ultrasound scans.

HIV test (for human immunodeficiency virus) Anyone who is at risk can ask to be tested. This test is carried out only with your consent.

If you have the disease, any infections that you develop must be carefully treated. The risk of transmitting HIV to your baby can be reduced by taking certain precautions at birth, including delivery by Caesarean section; it is also not advisable to breastfeed.

Sickle cell test (for sickle cell anaemia) This test is necessary if you, or any of your ancestors, come from an area where sickle cell anaemia (or thalassaemia, see below) is widespread, especially Africa and the West Indies.

The test examines the type of haemoglobin in your red blood cells and detects the sickle cells. If sickle cell trait or disease is found, your partner should be tested as well. If he is positive, the baby is at risk of being born with the disease. An amniocentesis or cordocentesis test will confirm or rule out this possibility (see p. 56).

Haemoglobin electrophoresis test (for thalassaemia) This test is advisable if you, or any of your ancestors, come from Asia and parts of Africa. It identifies the different haemoglobins that denote thalassaemia disease. If this trait is discovered, the baby may develop the disease. You may also become anaemic and require iron and folic acid supplements.

ALPHA-FETOPROTEIN

This is a protein that is first produced by part of the embryo, and then later by the fetal liver. Doctors use AFP as an indicator of what is going on inside the uterus.

AFP is commonly found in varying amounts in your blood throughout pregnancy. Between 16–18 weeks, the levels are usually low, so if a blood test is performed (see Triple or Bart's Test, opposite) and the levels are 2–3 times higher than the average of a sample, it may indicate a neurological problem such as hydrocephalus.

However, the levels may be raised because of a multiple pregnancy, inaccurate dating of the pregnancy, abnormalities of the baby's kidneys or digestive tract, or if there is a threat of miscarriage. Therefore, an ultrasound scan (see p. 32) will be taken to check for multiple birth, or to confirm your dates in case your pregnancy is more advanced than you think.

If the ultrasound scan rules out either possibility, further blood tests will be performed, and then you will be offered amniocentesis (see p. 56).

An abnormally low level of alpha-fetoprotein may suggest that the fetus may have Down's syndrome and, again, you will be offered amniocentesis to confirm or rule out this diagnosis.

WHY A SCAN IS OFFERED

Scans are normally offered to check the baby's progress, but there are other occasions when an ultrasound scan will be useful:

• *As part of assessment for infertility.*

• *To identify abdominal conditions such as an ectopic pregnancy.*

• *If the doctors suspect an imminent miscarriage.*

• *To check for a multiple pregnancy.*

ULTRASOUND SCAN

With the aid of an ultrasound scan you can see a picture of your unborn baby. An ultrasound scan checks the baby's general well-being and position, and guides doctors when performing special tests and operations. Most women will be offered a scan at least once during their pregnancy. It is routinely performed between 20 and 22 weeks when the baby can be seen at various angles. If any problems are detected, repeat scans may be performed several times before the birth.

HOW IT WORKS

The process is based on a sonar device that reveals objects in fluid, which was first used by the US navy to detect submarines during World War II. A crystal inside a device called a transducer converts an electrical current into high-frequency soundwaves that are inaudible to the human ear. The soundwaves form a beam that penetrates the abdomen as the transducer is moved back and forth. The beam reflects off material in its path, and the transducer records these echoes. The echoes are converted into electrical signals, which produce an image that can be displayed on a television-like screen. The beam can only penetrate fluids and soft tissue such as the amniotic sac, kidneys and liver. It cannot pass through bone or register gas. An ultrasound scan is

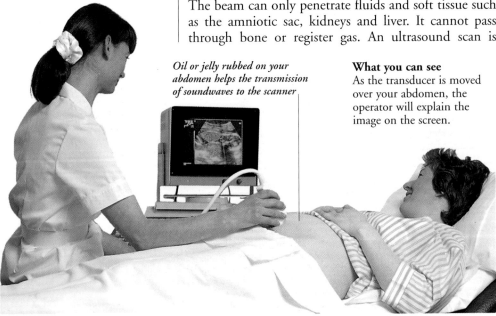

Oil or jelly rubbed on your abdomen helps the transmission of soundwaves to the scanner

What you can see
As the transducer is moved over your abdomen, the operator will explain the image on the screen.

increasingly used to assess threatened miscarriage; exclude ectopic pregnancies; during infertility treatments, such as IVF; and during fetal surgery.

YOUR FIRST SCAN

The sophisticated equipment used for an ultrasound scan may at first appear rather daunting, but don't be intimidated. The scan offers an exciting opportunity for you and your partner to see your baby for the very first time. You should be able to hear a heartbeat, and to distinguish the gentle movement of hands and feet, waving and kicking. The ultrasound operator will explain the image on the screen because some detail may be difficult to interpret. Some clinics will give you a print of the image of your baby as a memento. You may be asked to come back to repeat the scan because the scanner could not pick up the baby properly.

WHAT HAPPENS

Having a scan is painless, and usually lasts about 15 minutes. You may be asked to drink about half a litre (a pint) of water and not to urinate before arriving at the clinic. This can be uncomfortable, but a full bladder will provide a clearer picture of your baby. You may be asked to remove some clothes and put on a hospital robe before lying on a bed beside the scanner. As the transducer is passed over your abdomen, the image appears on the screen, and you can enjoy your first view of your baby.

WHAT IT SHOWS ABOUT YOUR BABY

A routine scan will reveal if your baby is healthy, and it may be used for other reasons during your pregnancy:

• *To check the baby's location and development of the placenta.*

• *To check on the growth rate of the baby, particularly when the date of conception is uncertain.*

• *To discover if the baby is ready to be born, if overdue.*

• *To confirm that your baby is in the usual head-down position, and not bottom-down, after week 38.*

• *To exclude certain fetal abnormalities, such as spina bifida.*

• *To assist in any operations performed on the baby while still in the uterus.*

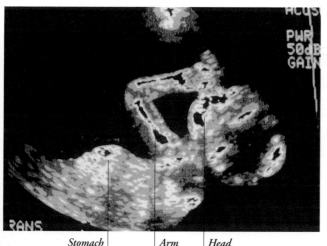

Stomach | Arm | Head

Baby at 22 weeks
An ultrasound scan will clearly show your baby's shape, his position, and whether you are expecting more than one. This portrait shows the baby in his mother's uterus. The baby floats and moves about continuously in the amniotic sac performing various activities: sucking his thumb, yawning, blinking, hiccupping and urinating.

NUCHAL SCAN

The picture below is the scan of a normal baby. The dotted lines indicate where the neck pad would be thicker in a baby that is likely to have Down's syndrome, heart defects or chromosomal abnormalities.

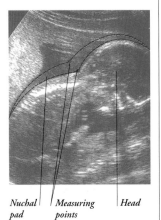

Nuchal | Measuring | Head
pad | points |

IS IT SAFE?

Unlike an X-ray, ultrasound scanning poses no known risk to the fetus. Questions have been raised about long-term effects, such as hearing impairment, caused by the impact of soundwaves. However, recent research seems to indicate that ultrasound is not harmful to the mother or the baby, because the waves are of a very low intensity, and so it is safe for the scan to be performed repeatedly. But, if you are worried, avoid having a scan before ten weeks, and do not have one unless it is necessary.

SPECIALIZED SCANS

Early on in your pregnancy, you may be asked to attend your hospital for a Nuchal or a Doppler scan. These are special ultrasound scans that are painless and are used to clarify possible problems, or when the baby seems not to be growing as much as expected. These are relatively new types of scan and may only be available at a larger hospital with a specialist unit.

Nuchal scan This scan is used at a very early stage (from 11 to 14 weeks) specifically to discover whether a baby might have Down's syndrome, or some other chromosomal problem. Unlike amniocentesis this is a non-invasive test and, while it cannot give a definitive answer, it is helpful in deciding whether further tests should be done.

During the scan the thickness (pad) of the back of the baby's neck ("nuchal" means neck) is measured (see left). In a Down's syndrome baby this neck pad is thicker than in a normal baby. A baby found to have such a pad will be tested further by amniocentesis (see p. 56), which can confirm or rule out the possibility of Down's syndrome.

Doppler scan The scan uses high-frequency sound waves of a different kind from those used in ordinary ultrasound scans. They are processed to reveal special wave forms, which can be used to show tiny movements within the growing fetus or placenta – for example, how the red blood cells are moving along blood vessels. This type of scan enables the scanner operator to see whether the placenta is working as it should, or if there is a possibility that the baby is not getting enough oxygen.

3

CHOOSING THE BIRTH YOU WANT

There are many decisions to make about what kind of

labour and birth you want. First, find out what is available

in your area then, after deciding whether you want a

hospital birth or a home birth and talking things over with

your partner, discuss your ideas with your doctor or

midwife. I recommend that you make a birth plan

outlining your preferences, because this will enable you to

be more assertive about the way your delivery is handled. It

is also advisable to attend childbirth classes, which will

provide both you and your partner with essential practical

training and moral support.

THE BRADLEY METHOD

This refinement of birth preparation was initiated by Dr. Robert Bradley and is also known as husband-coached childbirth.

The Bradley method teaches women to accept the pain, and to go with the flow under the guidance of the husband or partner, friend, or counsellor. The coach attends the antenatal classes with the mother, helps her with her exercise and breathing routine, and comforts, coaxes and coaches her through labour and delivery.

The failing of this method is that most women need to be distracted from pain in order to focus outside of themselves. Getting in touch with the pain can be totally overwhelming, making it more, not less, difficult to cope.

Each labour is completely unpredictable and your experience may be dissimilar to what you have prepared for. A woman often reacts to giving birth in a different way than she imagined. Also, some birth partners can become so enthusiastic about their coaching that they lose sight of the woman and her particular needs.

CHILDBIRTH PHILOSOPHERS

There have been a number of people who have influenced the way women and their carers approach birth today. Their teaching and ideas have altered antenatal and post-natal care, thus making childbirth an ever-evolving experience, and they have greatly affected the approach and procedures employed in childbirth in the West.

DR. GRANTLEY DICK-READ

Dr. Dick-Read was the first obstetrician to realize that fear of giving birth was one of the main causes of pain during labour, and he brought the principles of natural childbirth to the attention of not only the medical world, but to parents as well. He introduced proper education of mothers through antenatal classes and teaching, and also provided emotional support, in the idea of eliminating fear and tension. His teaching was so fundamental that it is now taken for granted by all centres, and there is no method of childbirth that does not rely on his ideas, which included breathing exercises, breathing control, and complete relaxation. Dr. Dick-Read's watchword was preparation – not only by getting information about childbirth, but also by seeking reassurance and sympathy.

FREDERICK LEBOYER

The Leboyer method of delivery works best if it's seen as an attempt to help people understand what the newborn baby sees, hears and feels. Leboyer was influenced by the psychiatrists Reich, Rank and Janov, who shared the belief that later problems in life stem from the process of birth. Leboyer's concern, therefore, is not primarily with the mother, but rather with the baby's experience of delivery.

In order to minimize the effects of birth, his book *Birth Without Violence* states that the birthing room should have soft lighting, and that noise and movement be kept to a minimum. Leboyer believes that immediate skin-to-skin contact is essential to calm the baby, and that she should be laid on her mother's stomach as soon as she is born. He suggests that the newborn should then be bathed in warm water as this is close to the internal environment of the uterus.

Not all of this fits in with the physiology of what actually occurs at birth. A baby needs the shock of feeling cool air on her skin to make her gasp and fill her lungs with her first breath: placing her in a warm liquid doesn't accomplish this kick-start. Many professionals say that there is no proof that Leboyer's theories work. However, it is only right that every baby be welcomed into the world with reverence, so even if you don't agree with all of Leboyer's theories, you can still be interested in a gentler birth.

DR. MICHEL ODENT

As a surgeon, Dr. Odent was extremely shocked when he first saw women on their backs with their feet held in stirrups, pushing their babies out against the force of gravity. This traditional delivery position meant that stronger, more painful contractions were needed to push the baby uphill, labour was slower and more exhausting, and there were more complications.

This led him to devise his own methods of childbirth, broadly based on traditional midwifery, at Pithiviers in France. Odent believes that, given the opportunity, women in labour return to a primitive biological state where they function at a new level of awareness and follow their basic instincts. He believes that endorphins, the body's natural narcotics, are responsible for this. Using his methods, Pithiviers has the lowest rate in France for episiotomy, forceps delivery and Caesarean section, and all interference is kept to a minimum.

SHEILA KITZINGER

A very highly respected birth practitioner, Kitzinger believes that birth is a very personal experience, and that the labouring mother should be an active "birth-giver", rather than a passive patient.

She believes that the maternity services must enable parents to have a real choice, whether that be a totally managed birth, a totally natural birth, or somewhere in-between, and that it's essential to respect parents' wishes. She also believes that birth is not an illness, and that professionals must not treat a labouring mother and her partner as patients, but as intelligent adults whose right it is to have the final say in decisions surrounding the birth of their baby.

THE LAMAZE METHOD

This method of psychological counselling was pioneered in Russia, and was then adopted in France by Dr. Lamaze.

Over 90% of women in Russia and 70% of French women are now taught variations of the Lamaze method. It has become equally popular in the United States, and still forms the basic teaching of the National Childbirth Trust in the UK.

Lamaze felt that no matter how relaxed a woman was, she almost certainly would experience some pain, and that she would have to cope with it. Following the reporting of Ivan Pavlov's research into stimulus-response conditioning in dogs, Lamaze saw the value of conditioned learning in helping women cope with the pain of childbirth.

The method has three mainstays. The first is that your fear of labour is reduced or eliminated by information and understanding. Second, you learn how to relax and become aware of your body, and therefore how to cope with pain. Third, you consciously use rhythmic breathing patterns through each contraction in order to distract your mind from the pain.

THOUGHTS ON CHILDBIRTH

Most of the influential birth philosophers (see p. 36) have been concerned with natural childbirth.

"Natural childbirth means normal physiological childbirth. When childbirth becomes associated with varying degrees of fear and therefore varying degrees of tension, it becomes in varying degrees unphysiological or pathological."

Grantley Dick-Read

"Doctors and midwives, once they have become aware of the ordeal it is to be born, will meet the young newcomer with more sensitivity, more intelligence, and more respect."

Frederick Leboyer

"Everywhere around us, we saw doctors increasing their use of drugs and artificial intervention, while we have kept intervention to an absolute minimum, and considered drugs unnecessary and harmful."

Michel Odent

"Childbirth is not primarily a medical process, but a psycho-sexual experience. It is not surprising that adapting your responses to the stimuli it presents should involve a subtle and delicate working together of mind and body."

Sheila Kitzinger

YOUR CHOICES IN CHILDBIRTH

Over the past few decades, women have been taking greater control of their own health. In many cases, members of the medical profession have responded enthusiastically to the changing desires and needs of women, and the "choices" in childbirth have never been greater, nor our wishes more paramount. Today, most of us ask to have our children more naturally, and this option should be available to all of us, whether the birth is at home or in hospital. But we shouldn't ignore the benefits a managed birth can provide, particularly when childbirth doesn't go as smoothly as expected.

THE MANAGED OR HIGH-TECH BIRTH

The modern managed or high-tech birth in hospital came out of a justified concern for the mother and baby, and from increased medical knowledge of the physiological aspects of birth. In a managed birth, labour is actively controlled so that it fits into what is perceived as being normal (this perception can differ, however, depending on the hospital and the obstetrician). A managed labour is the norm for most hospital births and it is essential for those women who have complications during pregnancy, labour or birth – if you have high blood pressure, for example, or an anticipated breech birth. In these situations, you'll have all your antenatal check-ups in hospital, which can mean that you are seen by different doctors and midwives at each visit, possibly leading to discontinuity of care.

In this setting, too, you are most likely to experience medical intervention involving some of the most modern procedures in obstetrics. With this kind of labour, epidural anaesthesia is literally on tap and electronic fetal monitoring is standard. Your attendants will notice very small changes in your baby's condition and may be pressured to act on such changes. Consequently, with this type of birth there are more inductions and Caesareans, and more frequent use of forceps.

Although these practices are beneficial to a percentage of births where intervention is needed, the routine use of them often cannot be justified by hard evidence. So women who want to have complete control over their deliveries may feel very strongly about their use. However, some women feel that a hospital setting makes childbirth the event they expect it to be, and they would feel cheated, nervous or even second-class if they didn't have an obstetrician in attendance with high-tech equipment close by.

NATURAL CHILDBIRTH

It seems a paradox that you have to request a natural birth but even today you may find that childbirth is still dominated by obstetricians and a few old-fashioned midwives. However, if you make your preferences known early, a natural birth can be arranged.

It is reasonable for women to want to have a natural birth in which there is no fear because the whole process of birth and delivery is familiar; where there is no unnecessary medical intervention; where there is a calm, homely atmosphere; where mothers are allowed to do anything they desire – to take up any positions that are most comfortable; and not be under pressure to take pain-relieving drugs. Female bodies are well designed for giving birth; all the soft tissues of the birth passage can open up so that a baby is gently squeezed out. But breathing and relaxation techniques can make birth even easier to manage, and a number of natural childbirth philosophies advocate these techniques.

Although there are individual differences, all birth philosophies share one common aim – to enable women to give birth in the way they want. They emphasize the need for intense concentration on breathing patterns and the learned ability to relax your body at will. The best way to experience a totally natural birth is in a dedicated centre or at home.

HOME BIRTH

In many countries healthy women can opt for a home delivery if their pregnancy has been straightforward. In the UK it is more difficult. When considering a home birth, most doctors would like you to have had one normal child by a normal delivery, before agreeing to a home birth for a second baby. Arranging a home birth can be difficult (see right), and you must be very sure that it is the best option for you. Keep an open mind about transferring to hospital if things do not progress well during labour.

ARE HOME BIRTHS SAFE?

A planned home birth can be one of the safest ways you can give birth.

A recent British report has concluded that although 94% of all births take place in hospitals, they are no safer, and may be less safe, than home births.

In Australia, a study of 3,400 home births found that there was a lower perinatal mortality rate, and less need for Caesareans, forceps and suturing for an episiotomy or a tear, than in hospital deliveries. The mothers were not all "low risk": the group included 15 multiple births, breech deliveries, women who had had Caesareans, and women with previous stillbirths. The group as a whole was older than the national average.

PLANNING A HOME BIRTH

Arranging a home birth isn't always straightforward, but it's worthwhile trying.

- *Visit your doctor and request a home birth.*

- *If your doctor agrees, arrange antenatal visits.*

- *If your doctor says no, find a midwife by contacting your hospital or the Independent Midwives' Association (see Useful Addresses).*

- *Arrange antenatal visits as usual with your new carer.*

YOUR HOME
BIRTH

At home, pre-labour will shift imperceptibly into full labour, without changes in location or your attendants.

- *You will remain in familiar surroundings with no need to travel while in labour.*

- *Once notified, your midwife will come to your house and stay with you throughout.*

- *You will be free to move around, and take up any position that feels comfortable.*

- *You will be encouraged to take your own time during labour.*

- *Your membranes are usually allowed to rupture spontaneously.*

- *You will be encouraged to seek relief of pain without drugs, although gas and oxygen, and pethidine are usually available.*

- *Your midwife will try hard to give your vagina time to stretch, so avoiding a tear and the need for an episiotomy.*

- *Your partner and family can be an integral part of the birth.*

- *You will have your baby with you at all times.*

- *After the birth you will be free to celebrate as you choose.*

HOME OR HOSPITAL?

The main difference between a home and a hospital birth is that at home you are the team captain, and everyone else is there to support you. You will have the same midwife throughout and you will not be separated from your baby or your partner afterwards. On the other hand, if you are in hospital and should anything go wrong, emergency medical assistance is immediately available.

HOME BIRTH

During the early stages of labour, you will probably find it is more comfortable if you move around. Once labour has become established, you or your partner should telephone the midwife if she isn't already on her way, as well as any other people whom you want to be present.

When the midwife arrives Your midwife will ask about your progress and examine you. She will be with you throughout labour, and she will monitor the baby every five minutes with a sonicaid (see p. 61). With your partner she will encourage you and help you into the most comfortable positions; some pain relief will be available if you need it.

Giving birth As the baby is being born, you will probably find it helpful to squat. Your partner may "catch" the baby before placing him onto your abdomen. His cord will be clamped and cut once it has stopped pulsating, then he will be quickly checked over, and the midwife will help you deliver the placenta. A little later, the baby will be given a thorough examination and weighed in a spring scale. You will be cleaned up and, if necessary, sutured. Then you can become acquainted with your new family member.

There are certain clear advantages to having your baby at home, such as the security of being in familiar surroundings with all the privacy you require. Your partner can play an integral part in the birth and your other children may also be present. You will avoid routine medical intervention. At home you don't have to perform according to preconceived medical ideas of what is normal. Disadvantages include the fact that if something does go seriously wrong, you will have to go into hospital.

HOSPITAL BIRTH

Most babies are born in hospital. Although more women are choosing to have babies at home, the majority of women, encouraged by their medical advisers or their own predilections, will give birth in hospital.

WHAT TO EXPECT

The unfamiliarity of hospital surroundings can add to the drama of the occasion, but with a birth partner to give you support and your own comfort aids such as music, the experience should be more pleasurable.

These days, most hospitals are more relaxed about making you feel comfortable. Trading your own clothes for a hospital gown can be de-personalizing so, if this bothers you, find out beforehand if you can wear your own nightdress or a tee-shirt. If you normally wear contact lenses, tell the hospital because they may prefer you to wear spectacles during the delivery.

After admission On arrival, your doctor or midwife will ask you about the progress of labour; examine your abdomen to confirm the situation; the baby's position will be felt and the baby's heart checked. You'll be given an internal examination to see how far your cervix has dilated. Fetal monitoring equipment may be set up. It can be awkward to move around once the equipment is attached so you may have to stay in one place.

Giving birth If you wish to manage without drugs for as long as possible during labour, the midwives will be happy to help you cope by using other methods. Drug relief such as epidural anaesthesia is usually available.

If you are in any danger of tearing, an episiotomy (an incision that helps deliver the baby's head) may be performed as the head is crowning. Your baby will be delivered on to your abdomen and, while you take your first look at each other, you will be given an injection into your thigh so that your uterus will contract, thus helping to expel the placenta. Your baby will then be checked over and weighed while you are cleaned up. If you need stitches, you are usually sutured by the midwife at this point, although in some hospitals you may have to wait for a doctor to do this.

YOUR HOSPITAL BIRTH

Your experience of giving birth will vary depending on your choice of hospital and professional attendants (see p. 22), but will probably include the following procedures. If you wish your labour to be different, talk to your doctor or midwife, or bring a birth plan (see p. 52).

- *You will probably travel to hospital while you are in labour.*

- *You will go through brief hospital admission procedures.*

- *If necessary, your membranes may be ruptured and fetal monitoring equipment set up.*

- *If labour slows down, or stops, you will probably be given Syntocinon (see p. 66) in order to stimulate contractions.*

- *Pain-relieving drugs of different types, including epidural anaesthesia, will usually be available.*

- *Your birth partner will usually be allowed to stay with you during labour and the birth.*

- *You will probably be attended by shifts of different midwives and doctors, especially if you are in labour into the night.*

- *You will probably be given an injection to help you deliver the placenta.*

- *You will be given your baby to hold immediately after the birth and encouraged to start breastfeeding.*

YOUR
CONSIDERATIONS

*There are many things that
you need to think about or
investigate when you are
selecting a hospital in which
to give birth. Here are some
questions to ask yourself, or
others, before you decide.*

• *What sort of birth do I
want – active, natural or
managed?*

• *What birth facilities are on
offer in my area?*

• *Am I prepared, or able, to
travel for antenatal care? Can
it be provided by my doctor?*

• *What sort of reputations do
the hospitals in my area have?*

• *What are the staff at the
different hospitals actually
like? What are their views on
labour and birth? Do I agree
with them?*

• *Do I want a special care
baby unit to be immediately
available?*

• *How long do I want to be
in hospital for, and what sort
of rooming-in facilities are
available to me?*

• *Do I want to feed my baby
whenever and however I feel
like it without pressure?*

• *Do I want my baby with me
at night? All night?*

• *What are the visiting hours?*

• *Can my partner (and
children) be with me whenever
I want?*

• *Can my partner stay with me
the first night after the birth?*

SELECTING A HOSPITAL

Information about the hospitals in your area is available
from your doctor, antenatal clinic, social worker, friends
and acquaintances. However, the only way to find out
what a hospital can offer you and whether you feel that
it is right for you, is to visit it and to ask questions. Take
a list of questions with you and make sure you get satisfactory answers so that you can come to a confident and
wholehearted decision.

WHICH HOSPITAL

There are various kinds of hospitals, most of which
provide maternity care. The most modern facilities are
found in teaching hospitals, where doctors are always on
duty, so if you run into any complications, one will attend
you. As a rule, doctors at teaching hospitals are usually
more experienced in dealing with complicated births. The
smaller community hospitals tend to be more friendly and
flexible. There is much less red tape because there are
fewer staff and fewer patients; it's easier to meet the people
who can help you, and there's no doubt that you will be
able to arrange a more personalized childbirth.

VISIT THE HOSPITAL

To help you make your choice, the first thing to do is
visit one or more hospitals with your birth assistant.
There may a formal maternity tour, often as part of the
hospital's antenatal classes, but if not, ask for a personal
tour accompanied by a member of staff who knows the
hospital well. If the hospital will not allow you to see
the facilities, ask questions. If they're rigid in their
approach to visitors, they are likely to be equally rigid in
their approach to maternity care.

THE HOSPITAL'S PROCEDURES

Once you have decided, it is a good idea to visit the
hospital of your choice again so that you can meet
the staff who will be looking after you, and become
familiar with the delivery room and other facilities. If, after
discussion with the staff, you find that your hospital is not
able to live up to your expectations, remember that a
hospital is there to serve you, and you do have the right to
refuse certain procedures. If the hospital is unwilling to

listen to your point of view, you can arrange for a transfer to a different one, or opt for another type of care such as that provided by a family-oriented hospital (see below).

If, however, your midwife is part of the Domino or team midwife schemes (see p. 23), she will come into the hospital with you and deliver your baby there; the hospital staff are only rarely involved. If all goes well, you are discharged within a few hours and need have little to do with the hospital's procedures.

BIRTHING ROOMS

Quite a few hospitals now have birthing rooms that are unclinical and more like your own home, with comfortable chairs, low lighting, soft music, piles of cushions on which you can arrange yourself and even drinks and snacks in case you are thirsty or hungry.

The whole aim of a birthing room is to help the mother relax, overcome fears and relieve tension. A normal routine prior to birth makes for a normal delivery, and once you're in a birthing room you will not be moved unless an emergency occurs that requires immediate attention. This method prevents uncomfortable breaks with a jarring change of movement, mood and surroundings. It's not necessary to lie down to have your baby, or to be surrounded by rather intimidating technological paraphernalia. In a birthing room you can take up whatever position feels comfortable to give birth to your baby.

For many women, a birthing room provides the ideal compromise between a home and a hospital birth because it provides surroundings and facilities similar to those at home, but emergency expertise and equipment are available if the need arises.

MATERNITY CARE UNITS

Family-oriented maternity care is offered by some of the more progressive hospitals and larger medical centres. It is a philosophy aimed at nurturing the family unit during labour, delivery and after birth. It should offer the optional elimination of certain routine procedures and the addition of others such as low lighting during delivery, non-separation of parents and baby unless medically necessary, rooming in and early discharge. However, this varies from hospital to hospital and you'll have to visit the unit to discuss your options with the staff.

WHAT TO ASK THE HOSPITAL

Once you have chosen a hospital, find out as much as you can by asking questions.

- *Will I be able to wear my own clothes and personal effects (rings, contact lenses and spectacles)?*

- *Can my partner or friend stay with me throughout? Will they ever be asked to leave?*

- *Will I be able to move around freely during labour, and give birth in any position I choose?*

- *Will I be able to have the same carers throughout labour?*

- *Can I bring in my own midwife to attend to me throughout labour?*

- *Does the hospital have a birthing room? Are beanbags, birthing chairs and stools provided?*

- *Does the hospital offer birthing pools? If not, will I be able to use a hired one?*

- *What is the hospital policy on pain relief, routine electronic monitoring and induction?*

- *What kind of pain relief is available? Is this at all times?*

- *Will I be able to eat and drink if I want to?*

- *What is the hospital policy on procedures such as episiotomies, Caesareans and the expulsion of the placenta?*

- *What is the hospital policy on separation of parents and child in the first hour or later?*

Although you can make most of your preparations well in advance, you will still have a few things to take care of.

When you go into labour you should:

- *Call your midwife.*
- *Make contact with your partner or birth assistant.*
- *Get in touch with whoever is going to care for your other children, if it is not your partner.*
- *Check that the room is ready.*
- *Check that your labour aids are conveniently available.*
- *Have a hot, sweet drink and some toast to give you energy.*

Advance preparation
To avoid a last-minute panic, make a list of everything you need well in advance.

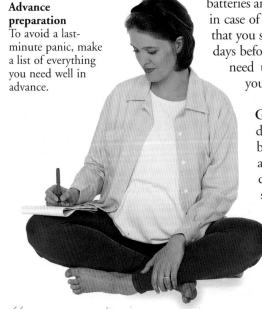

PREPARING FOR A HOME BIRTH

When you opt for a home birth, your midwife will give you detailed advice on the preparations you need to make. Think about what you will need for a home birth about four weeks in advance of your due date so that you do not have to rush around getting everything organized at the last minute, and you are at least partly prepared if your baby comes early.

YOUR BIRTHING ROOM

Your bedroom, or whichever room you intend to give birth in, should be arranged so that it is quiet, warm, convenient and comfortable for you. Put the bed at right angles to the wall, with plenty of space on each side so that the midwife has easy access.

Facilities for your midwife Ideally, provide your midwife with a small side table or a tea trolley next to the bed on which to put her instruments and other equipment, although a couple of tea trays will do. She will also need a bright, adjustable reading lamp so that she can direct light on to your perineum. A flashlight (with spare batteries and bulb) would be useful to have at hand in case of a power cut. You should also make sure that you stock up on snacks and drinks in the few days before you are due. Remember that you will need to provide food for your midwife and your birth attendant.

Getting the room ready Whether you deliver your baby on to the floor or the bed, the area below and immediately around you will need to be protected during the birth. Have some old clean sheets, towels or plastic sheeting available so that they can be put down when the time comes. Plastic sheeting is available from your local builders' merchant, although an old shower curtain or plastic tablecloth would be fine to use instead.

WHEN LABOUR HAS BEGUN

You can be sure labour has begun when your contractions are coming every 15 minutes or less, they are about one minute long, and don't die away when you move around. This is the time to telephone your midwife. It is common for first labours to take a while to get going so, although your midwife will want to know that things have started happening, she is likely to advise you to try and relax and get some rest until you are in full labour because it is important to conserve your energy. All independent midwives are usually contactable by radiopagers, so it is easy to keep in touch. Contact your birth partner if he or she is not already with you. You also need to make arrangements for someone to look after any other children you have.

Final preparations Make sure everything you and the midwife will need for the birth and immediately afterwards is prepared and ready to hand – including bowls for washing, a bedpan (or a clean bucket), clean towels and large plastic bags for the soiled dressings. Then put out a clean nightdress or large tee-shirt for yourself, air the baby's clothes and prepare the baby's cot. Once your midwife and birth attendant have arrived, take the telephone off the hook.

Your midwife's equipment The delivery equipment she brings will include a sphygmomanometer to take blood pressure; sonicaid to listen to the baby's heart; Entonox (gas and oxygen) cylinder; urine-testing sticks; local anaesthetic and syringes; scissors; suture material; mucus extractor; resuscitation equipment; intravenous equipment, in case of bleeding; and Syntometrine. If you wish to have pain-relieving drugs such as pethidine, she will give you a prescription to collect it in advance.

Unexpected hospitalization A home birth is completely safe but there can be complications. If a serious problem arises and you have to go into hospital to give birth, your midwife or doctor will accompany you. Being unable to have your baby at home, after all your preparation and anticipation, can be bitterly disappointing, but if you and your partner consider and discuss the possibility in advance it will be easier to cope with if it happens.

WHEN A HOME BIRTH IS INADVISABLE

Normally, it is as safe to give birth at home as it is in a hospital, but in certain circumstances a hospital birth is your only option.

There are a number of factors that can make a hospital birth necessary. Some, such as diabetes, will mean that you have to plan on a hospital delivery; others, which occur suddenly, such as placental abruption, will mean that you have to abandon your plans for a home birth and go immediately to hospital. The factors that rule out a home birth include:

- *When you have had complications in previous pregnancies.*

- *When your pelvis is too small for your baby's head to pass through it.*

- *When your baby is presenting in the breech position.*

- *When you have a medical problem that puts you, your baby, or both of you at risk, such as high blood pressure, anaemia, diabetes, excess amniotic fluid, active herpes, placenta praevia, placental abruption and pre-eclampsia.*

- *When you have a multiple pregnancy.*

- *When your baby is premature.*

- *When your pregnancy goes well beyond your estimated delivery date.*

CHILDBIRTH TEACHERS

You'll probably choose a childbirth teacher or class fairly early in your pregnancy; make plans to start classes in your seventh month or earlier. In some cases, you may have to book a place.

Both the quality and approach of classes can vary – some are tightly structured, with little question-and-answer time, others allow plenty of time to practise techniques. Some depend mainly on lectures, others on class participation. The teacher is very often the determining factor, so if you can, check with other couples you know have attended classes before you make your final choice.

Try to select a teacher whose philosophy of birth fits in with the type of birth you'd like to have. Conflicts and confusion can arise if what you learn in class does not accord with your later experience in hospital or at home.

Find out how many couples are taught in each class. Half a dozen couples is ideal, because you will receive plenty of attention from the teacher while being intimate with your fellow participants.

Most childbirth teachers will be very happy to talk to you about their approach – even if you are not yet attending childbirth classes.

CHILDBIRTH CLASSES

As an enthusiastic proponent of prepared childbirth, I believe that everyone can benefit from childbirth or parentcraft classes. These classes can be tremendously enjoyable. The camaraderie is wonderful and you may find that the other members of the group act as a substitute for your extended family as you exchange folklore; certainly they will make you feel less alone and isolated. It's a great benefit to be able to share feelings and experiences with people who are in the same position and it helps to relieve tension and anxiety. Strong personal bonds are often formed with others in the class that can be the basis of lasting friendships. It's important that your partner goes with you to these classes; most prospective fathers find them very useful.

TOPICS COVERED

Childbirth or parentcraft classes are particularly useful for first-time parents because they're designed to give you information that will make you both feel more confident. They work in three ways:

First, they cover the processes of pregnancy and birth, including female anatomy and physiology, and the changes that occur throughout pregnancy. This is done so you will have a clearer understanding of what is involved and why things are happening. Your teacher will also talk to you about the sort of medical procedures that you can expect, and why these will be done.

Second, the classes provide practical instruction in relaxation, breathing and exercise techniques (see p. 48) that will help you to control your labour, reduce pain and will also give you the confidence that only comes with being familiar with what's happening. Bear in mind that bodies, not brains, give birth, so anything that helps you tune into your body is going to be useful. Your partner should also learn how to give you a massage to help relieve your pain.

Third, your teacher will talk you through the stages of labour and birth, and aspects of postnatal recovery. You will be advised on breastfeeding, making up formula and bottlefeeding, and both you and your partner can practise bathing and dressing a baby and changing nappies. This will help you cope with the practicalities of babycare.

EXERCISE CLASSES

Doing exercises that strengthen the muscles used in childbirth often results in an easier delivery (see p. 48). Many hospitals offer antenatal classes that incorporate exercise and relaxation techniques, and there are independent organizations as well – some are even for specific types of birth. If you tell your instructor that you would like to have your baby in a standing or squatting position, for example, you will be given suitable exercises to help strengthen the muscles in your back, hips and legs.

TECHNIQUES FOR EASIER CHILDBIRTH

Studies have shown that taking childbirth classes shortens the length of labour. In one study, the average duration of labour for a group of women who had taken classes was 13.56 hours, compared with the average labour of 18.33 hours in the control group, which had no training. This is probably because knowing how to deal with pain produces a more relaxed labour. Strategies taught to deal with pain include the following:

Cognitive control You disassociate your mind from the pain by visualizing a pleasant scenario in which to experience the pain. In this way, you will be concentrating on the non-painful part of the sensation.

Systematic relaxation In order to increase your tolerance of pain, you are taught exercises to relax the various muscles of the body (see p. 49). In this way you will be able to isolate pain from the contracting uterus rather than allow it to pervade the rest of your body.

Hawthorne rehearsal You receive enhanced attention from a birth assistant. Psychological research has shown that the more attention given, the less pain you feel.

Systematic desensitization You gradually become more tolerant of pain. This often involves your coach pinching your leg very hard for you to practise coping with how painful a contraction can be. The pinching is repeated at each class, and by the end of the course you should be able tolerate pain for longer periods.

FATHER'S ROLE

In an antenatal class you may be able to show your partner for the first time just how central a role he is going to play.

Classes will make a supportive man a more effective birth assistant by familiarizing him with the processes of labour and delivery.

Some courses have father-only sessions where the men can talk freely about any problems or anxieties they have about the forthcoming event. A worried man should find security and support in the company of other fathers-to-be.

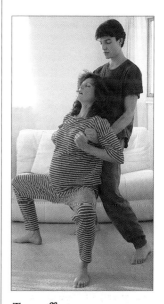

Team effort
Childbirth classes give a couple a unique opportunity to work as a team towards a common goal – the birth of their baby – and often this results in a special closeness.

YOUR PELVIC FLOOR

The pelvic floor muscles form a funnel that supports the uterus, bowel and bladder, and serve to close the entrances to the vagina, rectum and urethra.

During pregnancy, an increase in progesterone causes the muscles to soften and relax. To counter this there is an exercise you can do to keep the pelvic floor well toned and also prevent later problems.

Pull up and tense the muscles around your vagina and anus, as if you were stopping the flow of urine. Hold as long as you can without straining. Relax. Repeat 25 times a day.

You should restart this exercise as soon as you can after delivery to minimize the risk of prolapse. Early exercise will tone up the vagina for sexual intercourse too. Make this part of your daily routine.

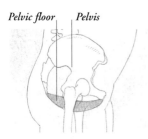

Pelvic floor   *Pelvis*

The pelvic floor

This consists of muscles and fibrous tissue suspended like a funnel from the pelvic bones. It forms a figure of eight around the urethra, vagina and anus. The layers of muscle are at their thickest at the perineum.

PREPARATION FOR LABOUR

As you approach your delivery date, your childbirth classes will help you prepare. You can also get yourself ready by practising pelvic floor exercises, breathing techniques and learning how to relax.

PELVIC FLOOR EXERCISES

During pregnancy and delivery your pelvic floor (see column, left) can be be stretched by the weight of the baby, which may cause discomfort and problems after the birth. You should perform pelvic floor exercises all through pregnancy and immediately after birth to keep the muscles of your pelvic floor firm and toned.

BREATHING TECHNIQUES

It's worth mastering breathing techniques because they are extremely useful during labour. In the first place, they give you a wonderful feeling of control over your body. But also, miraculously almost, breathing can increase your ability to cope with pain.

Any woman who wants at least to try natural childbirth can learn breathing exercises that may enable her to get through labour without resorting to painkillers or anesthetics. In addition, deep breathing will calm you, prevent you from becoming fearful and therefore help to conserve energy that you will need for bearing down. Each of the different levels of breathing is useful at a different point during labour. Make sure that your birth partner is familiar with them too, so that he or she can support and encourage you during labour.

Deep breathing The point of this kind of breathing is to fill the deepest point of your lungs with air so that your brain and the placenta receive plenty of oxygen. You should feel your ribcage lift upwards and outwards as you inhale. A trick I learned was to take in as much breath as I could and then, at the last moment, breathe in a little more. Then if you drop your shoulders, the elastic recoil of your lungs will expel the air slowly out. Concentrate on exhalation; it will help if your birth partner places their hands around your lower back and you let your ribs sink, with a sigh, into their cupped hands. This level of breathing is particularly helpful at the beginning and end of contractions.

Feather-light breathing I use this kind of breathing to prepare myself whenever I have to make a great physical effort. It's really just rapid panting and it serves at any time, but particularly during labour, to aerate the lungs very efficiently over a short space of time. In the transition period you need to do this to stop yourself bearing down before full dilation.

Take shallow breaths in and out so that you sound like a dog panting, using only the upper part of your lungs. After about 10–15 seconds of this, the body feels a blast of oxygen into the system. It's also very effective in eliminating carbon dioxide from your system. But it's main use in labour is to distract you – while you are panting you can't do much else. It primes you for action and, incidentally, stops you feeling pain as intensely – so it's excellent at the height of a contraction.

To prevent yourself from overbreathing, hold your breath for a count of five every 10–15 breaths. It is during this breath-holding time in stage two of labour that you would push.

Light breathing This kind of breathing uses the upper half of your lungs to the extent that you feel your shoulders and shoulder-blades rising. You concentrate very hard on breathing in through your mouth and throat with your lips apart and take short, sharp breaths. This level of breathing is useful at the height of a painful contraction. To practise, get your birth partner to place their hands on your upper back so that you get the feel of the movement.

WHY RELAXATION HELPS

The benefits of learning relaxation techniques are several: it enables you to conserve energy during pregnancy by resting *instantly* whenever you are tired during the day or evening. Even a few minutes of relaxation are refreshing and allow you to make the most of spare moments to replenish your energy. It is also useful during labour to be able to relax your body at will because this will help reduce tension and enhance your ability to tolerate pain.

RELAXATION TECHNIQUES

The benefit of learning to relax the muscles of your body in sequence is that you can isolate yourself from the uterus in labour, so that it alone is contracting, while none of your other muscles is tense.

The best way to isolate a group of muscles is to tense them, feel the tension then let go. Start by practising twice a day for 15–20 minutes in a comfortable position sitting or lying with your eyes closed. Speak to the muscles in your forehead first. Tense them and then let them relax. Work down your body in sequence – your eyes, cheeks, jaw, chin, neck, shoulders, arms, hands – down the body until your whole body feels heavy. A good test of how relaxed you are is if you can feel that whatever you're sitting or lying on is pushing back into your body.

Mental relaxation *This is achieved through the skill of physical relaxation. First clear your mind – my trick is to think of black velvet – and concentrate on calming your breathing. Cut down your rate of breathing by half. If any troublesome thoughts recur, stop them with a mental "no". Then think of the most tranquil scene you can imagine, and keep it in your mind's eye. Breathe deeply and slowly the entire time.*

FIT FOR PREGNANCY

By performing exercises, you will relieve the strain caused by your extra weight and strengthen important muscles. Practise these daily if possible, building repetitions gradually. Don't get overheated while exercising. Remember to drink plenty of water. Stop immediately if anything hurts, or if you feel sick, dizzy or breathless.

PELVIC TILT

Do pelvic tilt exercises to strengthen your lower back and abdominal muscles, so preventing bad posture and backache.

Upright position
With your feet resting flat on the floor, sit on a stool or chair. Rock your pelvis forward. Then pull in your stomach muscles and rock back on your hips. Release. Repeat this several times.

On all fours
Breathe in, then exhale and lift your back and pull in your stomach muscles, clenching your buttock muscles. Hold, then release and return your back to a level position, holding your stomach muscles firm. Repeat this several times.

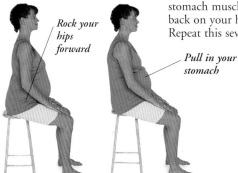

Rock your hips forward

Pull in your stomach

Pull in your stomach muscles

HIPS AND TRUNK
Your mobility can be increased by twisting and circling exercises; these loosen the trunk area. You may also find the hip circling movement (left) is especially helpful during the first stage of labour to relieve backache.

Circling your hips
Place your feet apart and have your knees slightly bent, with hands on hips. Slowly circle your hips around in one direction five to ten times; then repeat in the other direction.

Twisting
Sit with your feet flat on the floor and your knees apart. Raise your arms to chest level and twist your upper body to one side as far as you can, then to the other. Repeat.

Keep your arms at chest level

Twist to the left then to the right

Keep your knees slightly bent

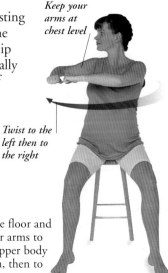

LEG STRETCHES

During pregnancy, your legs have to carry a lot of extra weight, so it's important to stretch and strengthen the muscles. These exercises will also improve the circulation in your legs.

Do not arch your back

Exercise to strengthen legs

Rest against a wall with your feet apart. Slowly bend your legs until you feel some pull on your thigh muscles but before you feel uncomfortable. Stay in this position for a count of 20, then stand up.

Straighten the back leg as you bend the front knee

Slowly bend your knees as far as you can

Stretching calf muscles

Facing a wall, bend your elbows and lean against the wall, with your weight on your forearms. Place one foot behind the other, ensuring that both feet point at the wall. As you bend one knee, stretch the rear calf muscle. Hold, then release and repeat with the other leg.

FEET AND ANKLES

Pregnancy hormones relax the walls of the veins, which slows the blood to the heart and can cause varicose veins and swollen ankles and legs. Do these exercises regularly to stimulate the circulation.

Foot exercises

Flex one foot up and down from the ankle, but do not point the toes (or you may get cramp). Repeat with the other foot. Do this ten to 20 times per foot at least twice a day.

If you find sitting on the floor in this position difficult, sit on a chair

Do not point your toes

Circle the feet

Gently circle your feet ten times one way and again the other way. Remember to keep your toes relaxed.

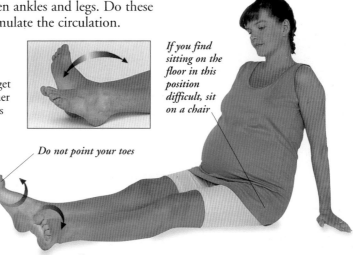

COVERING YOUR ALTERNATIVES

Although you will make your plan according to the kind of birth you would like to have, it is a good idea to have another one on stand-by.

This alternative plan can set out the procedures that you would prefer to be followed should complications arise. On rare occasions, labour may become unexpectedly prolonged or difficult, or the baby may need special attention. By considering all the possibilities, you enable your birth attendants to take care of any situation as you would wish.

YOUR BIRTH PLAN

Making a plan of your baby's birth will help to ensure you are actively involved in the way he is born. By carefully considering all your ideas and preferences, and by discussing them with your partner and birth attendants, you will be able to establish a bond of trust and create a happier and more comfortable labour.

A CONSENSUS PLAN

Think about the issues that are important to you and then find out whether what you want is feasible (see pp. 42 and 54). There is no point in making a plan that cannot be used once you are in labour. Discuss your ideas with your GP early in your pregnancy so that he or she can refer you to the consultant obstetrician most likely to accord with your wishes. You should make specific enquiries about the routines followed where you intend to give birth, as some hospitals will not be able to meet your requirements. Also discuss your ideas with your midwife, antenatal teacher, and other members of your antenatal team as they will be able to advise you about the kinds of experiences mothers have had in local hospitals and with particular doctors.

Hospital response   Your hospital team may be pleased to see how well you have prepared yourself for the labour and encourage your full participation. Some mothers experience negativity from hospital staff on the grounds that a birth plan interferes with their standard practices. Don't be intimidated – just remember your baby and the way in which you give birth are your responsibility.

Working together   Co-operation is an important feature of the birth plan. By working it out in detail with all concerned, you should be able to alleviate any anxieties and feel more in control of your baby's birth. Make sure, too, that staff know of any alternative plan (see column, left). Try to maintain a friendly relationship with your professional attendants as they are not bound to follow your wishes. Give a copy of the plan to your midwife or the hospital team; a copy should also be placed with your hospital records. This is important if you are attended in labour by someone who doesn't know your wishes.

Thank you for all the information that you have provided in the antenatal classes and at the childbirth classes. I have thought carefully about how I would like my labour and delivery to be.

My partner, John, will be my companion during labour. He has attended childbirth classes with me.

I understand that electronic fetal monitoring is routinely used and I am happy for this to be done.

If I need pain relief I would prefer an epidural, with as low an epidural dose as possible so that I still have feeling in my legs and am aware of contractions. I would prefer for it to wear off for the second stage, as I would like to push out the baby myself.

If everything goes well and I do not need pain relief, I would prefer to be able to walk around and give birth using a birthing stool, which I will provide myself.

If I have to have a Caesarean section I would like my partner to be with me throughout the operation.

I intend to breastfeed on demand and want the baby to sleep next to me if possible.

Jenny Lewis

I am looking forward to coming into Central Hospital. I would like to record a few points about the birth as the midwives have suggested. They are:

Support person	I will be accompanied by my sister, Sarah.
Shaving and enemas	I would prefer not to be shaved or to have an enema.
Monitoring	I would prefer to be monitored by a sonicaid.
Positions	I will probably want to deliver the baby in a semi-upright position, as this is how I had my other two babies.
Pain relief	It is likely that I will need gas and air, as I did last time.
Episiotomy	I would prefer not to be cut if it can be avoided. I would welcome help in order to help prevent it.

Paula Bell

Presenting your birth plan

These two examples of a birth plan outline different choices of birth – there are many variations. The plan may be laid out as a list, a letter or a document. It can be typed or hand-written. Remember to add your name and address and/or hospital number if you have one. Make a note on your birth plan of any special needs, such as diet, for example, which may be applicable during your time in hospital.

BIRTH PLAN QUESTIONS

Before it's possible to express preferences about the way you and your partner would like your birth to be conducted, you have to be familiar with the routine of the labour ward you have chosen. You will, of course, visit the hospital and talk to the staff about your preferences. It may be difficult to know where to start, so I suggest you draw up a list of questions for your carers before you go. Then write out your plan, working through labour systematically:

- How many birth partners am I allowed?
- If I have a Caesarean section, can my birth attendants come with me to the operating room?
- Will labour be induced artificially after the due date?
- Can I walk around, eat and drink during labour?
- Will I always be attended by a midwife I know?
- If there is a change of staff, will my new midwife be told of my birth plan?
- Does a doctor have to be present?
- Can I and my partner decide when and what kind of pain relief is administered?
- Does the hospital have epidural anaesthesia if I want it, available round the clock?
- Are there TENS machines available for hire?
- Is a water birth possible?
- Can I stand or squat to deliver my baby?
- Can I be given enough time to deliver the head so that I don't need an episiotomy?
- Are episiotomies often done under a local anaesthetic?
- Can I see my baby's head being delivered?
- Can I deliver the rest of my baby myself?
- Can we be left alone with the baby?
- Will my placenta be delivered naturally or with an injection of Syntometrine?
- Who stitches episiotomies – the midwife, or must I wait for a doctor to come?
- When can I go home?

WHEN DO I WRITE IT?

Although you will probably think about the issues involved from early on in your pregnancy, you don't need to finalize your plans until the eighth month.

CHAPTER 4

SPECIAL PROCEDURES

Check-ups and investigations will be carried out throughout your pregnancy and if a problem is suspected, special tests will enable your doctor to rule out or confirm whether the baby has been affected. Many disorders can now be detected with these invasive tests: chromosomal disorders such as Down's syndrome, for example, and genetically linked disorders such as haemophilia and cystic fibrosis. Mothers with serious conditions such as diabetes or Rhesus incompatibility will have special care throughout their pregnancies. If you go beyond your estimated delivery date, you will be closely monitored to ensure that all is well.

SPECIAL TESTS

If your doctor suspects that there is a problem that cannot be detected by routine tests, or if you have a family history of a particular disorder, you will be offered further, more specific tests. Apart from enabling doctors to check for various complications, they can perform two useful services for you and your partner: they can be reassuring and give you and your baby a clean bill of health and they may provide you with information that may cause you to question whether your pregnancy should proceed. Before making any decision, please have full discussions with your doctor about the tests and results and take advantage of the counsellors who are there to help you.

AMNIOCENTESIS

Amniotic fluid contains cells from the baby's skin and other organs which provide clues to his condition. Amniocentesis is the simple procedure that withdraws this fluid from the uterus.

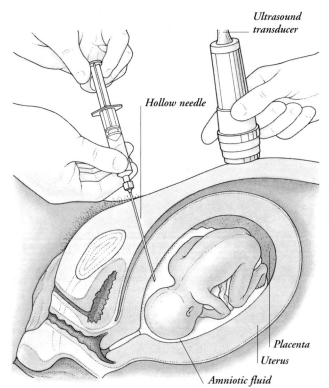

Ultrasound transducer

Hollow needle

Placenta

Uterus

Amniotic fluid

Amniocentesis
Amniotic fluid is extracted only after an ultrasound scan has determined the position of the fetus and the placenta. Using ultrasound, the doctor passes a needle through the abdominal wall, which has been numbed with local anaesthetic, and into the uterus. A small amount of amniotic fluid is withdrawn.

Why is it done? You will be offered an amniocentesis if you have a family history of Down's syndrome or if you are over the age of 35, when the risk of chromosomal abnormalities (such as Down's) is slightly higher, particularly if your blood tests have revealed a very low level of alpha-fetoprotein (see p. 31). In addition, amniocentesis can reveal other important information if there is already cause for concern. The test shows:

• The sex of the baby: fetal skin cells accumulate in the amniotic fluid. Under the microscope, these cells reveal the baby's sex. In genetically-linked disorders such as haemophilia, a male child has a 50 percent chance of being affected.

• The age of the baby: the lecithin/sphingomyelin (L/S) ratio in the fluid is measured. This ratio allows doctors to assess the maturity of the lungs, which is an indication of fetal age.

• The chemical composition of the fluid: this can reveal metabolic disorders caused by missing or defective enzymes.

• The bilirubin content of the fluid: this helps determine if a Rhesus-positive baby needs an intrauterine blood transfusion.

• The amount of oxygen the baby is getting: gases dissolved in the amniotic fluid are measured, revealing whether the baby is at risk from lack of oxygen.

• Acidity of the fluid is another indication of fetal distress, often caused by inadequate oxygen flow to the baby.

• The chromosome count: determined by examining discarded cells. Deviation from the normal chromosomal structure may mean that the baby will be handicapped in some way.

How is it done? Amniocentesis is usually performed between 14 and 20 weeks, although it can be done a little earlier. A hollow needle is inserted into the amniotic sac through the front of the abdominal wall, and about 14 grams (½ ounce) is usually withdrawn. This is then spun in a centrifuge to separate the cells shed by the baby from the rest of the liquid. The cells are cultured for about two to five weeks, and therefore the results take some time. The risk of the procedure inducing a miscarriage in early pregnancy is about one in 200.

CHORIONIC VILLUS SAMPLING (CVS)

The chorionic villi are finger-like outgrowths of the chorion, which form the baby's side of the placenta; they are genetically identical to the fetus. As they develop earlier than the amniotic fluid, examining a sample of chorionic villi will provide information about your baby's genes and chromosomes some weeks before amniocentesis is possible.

Chorionic villi

Amniotic sac

Ultrasound transducer

Fetus | Uterus

Hollow needle

Chorionic sampling
A small amount of chorion (placental tissue) is taken from the uterus through the cervix with the aid of a hollow needle (catheter).

Why is it done? The most important group of mothers needing CVS are those at risk of having a Down's syndrome baby. An abnormality of haemoglobin, such as sickle-cell disease or thalassemia, can be diagnosed with CVS. Hereditary metabolic disorders are fortunately rare, but if a family is affected, the frequency may be as high as one in four. The basic defect is an enzyme deficiency, and direct enzyme analysis of the chorionic tissue will provide the diagnosis within two days. Single gene disorders, such as cystic fibrosis, haemophilia, Huntington's chorea, and muscular dystrophy, can be detected by microscopic analysis of chorionic villi.

How is it done? CVS is carried out under ultrasound control, usually between 10 and 12 weeks, before the amniotic sac completely fills the uterine cavity. For this procedure, one of two routes is employed: the trans-cervical route or the trans-abdominal route.

For the trans-cervical route (see diagram, left), a plastic or metal hollow needle (catheter) is introduced through the cervical canal into the outside edge of the placenta. A small amount of chorionic villi tissue is removed. The trans-abdominal procedure is similar to that of amniocentesis (see p. 56), but the sample is taken from the placental tissue instead of the amniotic fluid.

The risk of miscarriage following CVS is about two percent higher than the spontaneous miscarriage rate. The advantage of CVS is that it can be performed earlier in pregnancy than amniocentesis.

UMBILICAL VEIN SAMPLING (CORDOCENTESIS)

This procedure is carried out at about 20 weeks or later, often following the ultrasound scan at this time. It is used to examine the constituents of the baby's blood and, in the case of fetal anaemia, to determine if an intrauterine blood transfusion is necessary. It is also vital in four other situations.

Detecting infection Rubella (German measles), toxoplasmosis and the herpes virus may be detected by performing a specific radio analysis of certain proteins that are present in the blood of the fetus.

Rhesus iso-immunization In cases of Rhesus incompatibility (see p. 62) the direct assessment of fetal haemoglobin is the best way to determine if the baby is coping or becoming anaemic, and whether an intrauterine blood transfusion (also done through the umbilical vein) needs to be carried out.

Chromosome count Analysis of certain white blood cells (fetal lymphocytes) will detect chromosomal abnormalities that are associated with Down's syndrome and other conditions. The results take a few days to come through.

Suspected growth retardation If the fetus is considered to be growth-retarded, cordocentesis may be used to measure the acidity or alkalinity of the blood, the amount of oxygen and carbon dioxide and the amount of bicarbonate in the blood. In addition, plasma levels of glucose can be estimated.

How is it done? Under ultrasonic control, a hollow needle is passed through the front wall of the abdomen and uterus into a blood vessel in the umbilical cord, about 1cm (½in) from where it emerges from the placenta. A small quantity of blood can then be removed for testing. It takes about a week for results.

The risk to the fetus appears to be about one to two percent. In theory, cordocentesis can replace any investigation currently undertaken on a blood sample.

OTHER TESTS FOR CHROMOSOMAL DEFECTS

Bart's or Triple test This is a screening blood test (see p. 30) that has been developed by St. Bartholomew's Hospital in London. A maternal blood sample is taken at 16 weeks to measure the levels of three substances: oestriol, human chorionic gonadotrophin and alpha-fetoprotein. The results can be assessed, along with your age, to predict the chance of your baby suffering from Down's syndrome. If the chances seem high, amniocentesis (see p. 56) is then offered. The Bart's test is not yet widely available, although you can request it.

Ultrasound scanning Recent research seems to indicate that Down's syndrome and other chromosomal defects can be identified by a special procedure using ultrasound scanning called a Nuchal scan (see p. 34). This investigates the size and shape of the neck pad at the back of the fetus' neck and may suggest that a defect may be present. If so, amniocentesis or CVS will be offered.

THE EFFECT OF YOUR AGE

Your age is an important factor in how your baby develops but it's just one of several factors that can affect the outcome of your pregnancy; your lifestyle and nutrition are much more important. However, the older you are when you become pregnant, the more likely you are to require special attention. You'll be asked questions to identify whether you have any problems and appropriate tests will be offered to rule out certain disorders (see below).

Down's syndrome Maternal age does seem to be an important factor in what causes Down's syndrome, although parents of any age can have a baby with this condition. As you can see from the graph (left), the risk of having a Down's baby rises with advancing maternal age, but isn't really significant until after 35 years of age. However, as a Down's baby is born every 2,000 births, and as most babies are born to women under 35 who do not undergo screening for Down's syndrome, there are more Down's babies born in the pre-35 age group than in the post-35 age group.

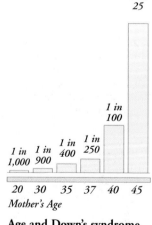

Age and Down's syndrome
The chart shows that the risk of having a Down's syndrome baby rises rapidly after 35 years of age.

FETAL HEART MONITORING

This is an efficient method of monitoring the well-being of the fetus during pregnancy. A healthy fetus that is receiving adequate supplies of oxygen and nutrients, will generally be more active than a malnourished, oxygen-starved fetus, and the heart rate will respond to stress more effectively.

Doctors and midwives use a hand-held monitor called a sonicaid to check the presence and rate of the heartbeat at every antenatal visit from week 14. This is a small portable instrument, which uses ultrasound, that is placed on your abdomen. The sonicaid also magnifies the sound so that you can listen to it.

The baby's heartbeat is much faster than your own (about 115 beats per minute compared with 75 beats per minute), and sounds just like a tiny galloping horse. When a healthy, active fetus moves, the heart rate accelerates by 15 beats per minute for 15 seconds. If your baby is distressed for any reason, the heart rate dips. Fetal heart monitoring is also useful during labour to detect signs of distress.

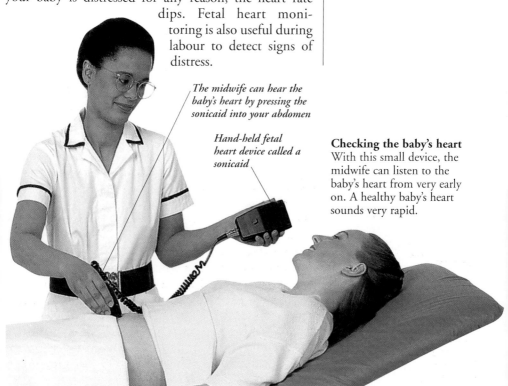

The midwife can hear the baby's heart by pressing the sonicaid into your abdomen

Hand-held fetal heart device called a sonicaid

Checking the baby's heart
With this small device, the midwife can listen to the baby's heart from very early on. A healthy baby's heart sounds very rapid.

ANTI-D (RHOGHAM) INJECTIONS

To prevent destructive antibodies from forming and attacking any subsequent babies, pregnant women who are Rhesus-negative need an anti-D (Rhogham) injection:

- *After delivery.*

- *After a miscarriage or an abortion.*

- *After chorionic villus sampling (CVS).*

- *After an amniocentesis or cordocentesis, especially if there is blood on the needle after it has been withdrawn from the uterus.*

RHESUS INCOMPATABILITY

About 85 percent of the population has a substance called the Rhesus factor in their red blood cells. These people are known as Rhesus positive. The remaining 15 percent, whose blood cells lack the Rhesus factor, are Rhesus negative. Rhesus positivity is always dominant; negativity will only exist when only negative genes are inherited. Being Rhesus negative does not affect you unless you are pregnant or need a blood transfusion.

AN INCOMPATIBLE MOTHER AND BABY

In pregnancies where the mother has Rhesus-negative blood and the baby Rhesus-positive (an incompatible pregnancy), the first pregnancy usually goes without a hitch. However, when fetal blood cells mix with maternal cells, for example, during delivery, the mother's blood becomes sensitized.

When the Rh factor from the baby's blood enters the mother's bloodstream, it acts as an antigen and stimulates production of anti-Rhesus-positive antibodies. These will attack and destroy the blood cells of her next Rhesus-positive (incompatible) baby. This causes haemolytic disease of the newborn and infants are affected with blood conditions ranging from mild jaundice to serious, possibly fatal, anaemia. Fetuses who develop the disease can often be saved by an intrauterine blood transfusion.

Not all Rh-negative women with Rh-positive babies become sensitized, but there is no way of predicting which women will. All of these women, therefore, are carefully monitored and given preventative injections in certain situations (see column, left) and after delivery.

CAREFUL MONITORING

The mother's blood will be monitored throughout her pregnancy. At each visit, she will have a special specimen of blood taken to examine for increasing levels of antibodies. Only if they increase beyond a certain point is the developing baby in any danger. If increasing antibodies are found, the mother will have an ultrasound scan at 18 weeks. This can check for the presence of fetal bilirubin (a by-product of red blood cell destruction) in the amniotic fluid.

In the third trimester, a direct test for the presence of bilirubin can be done by a process called cordocentesis (see p. 59). This test enables the doctors to assess the severity of the condition and determine whether blood transfusions are necessary.

If the antibody count remains low, the mother will not require further special care. However, if the count rises moderately, her baby may be induced early to prevent serious consequences. In this case, home birth is out of the question and she will need to deliver in a hospital.

Within 48 hours of delivery, the mother is injected intra-muscularly with anti-D (Rhogham) to help prevent the destructive antibodies from forming and attacking her next baby.

RHESUS DISEASE IN PREGNANCY

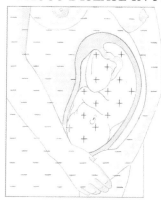

Rhesus disease only occurs when a woman who has Rhesus-negative blood (shown as red minus signs in the picture) is pregnant with a Rhesus-positive (the blue plus signs) baby. Most Rhesus-negative mothers carry their first babies without problems. If they then develop antibodies to Rhesus-positive blood (the green triangles), any subsequent babies could be at risk.

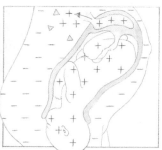

Mother is sensitized
Unless the mother is given an anti-D (Rhogham) injection within 48 hours of delivery, she may develop antibodies to Rhesus-positive blood.

A future pregnancy
These antibodies will mean that if she becomes pregnant with another Rhesus-positive baby, her antibodies may attack this baby's blood cells.

HOW THE BABY IS AFFECTED

The baby is likely to be fit and healthy, owing to the anti-D (Rhogham) injections and the special care given during pregnancy.

• Immediately after birth the baby will have a Coomb's test to reveal the presence of maternal anti-Rhesus-positive antibodies.

• If the baby is affected by Rh incompatibility, his levels of bilirubin will rise very quickly after birth because his liver has a poor ability to cope with it.

• The high level of bilirubin in his blood and tissues will make him look yellow. This can be treated by placing him under a "bili" light, which converts the bilirubin into a substance harmless to the brain.

IS MY BABY OVERDUE?

Only about five percent of all babies arrive on the date that they are expected. The estimated date of delivery (EDD) is only a statistical average, and studies have shown that as many as 40 percent of babies are born more than a week after the EDD. This 40 percent of "overdue" births breaks down as follows: 25 percent of babies are born in the 42nd week of pregnancy, 12 percent in the 43rd week, and three percent in the 44th week.

EVERY PREGNANCY IS DIFFERENT

One of the main difficulties in deciding whether a baby is actually overdue or not is that the precise date of conception in any particular pregnancy is unknown. Even if you have a regular menstrual cycle of 28 days (the standard on which the EDD chart is based), the date of ovulation is only known approximately. Apart from this uncertainty about the date of ovulation, every baby is different and it is therefore unrealistic to expect all babies to mature in precisely the same number of days. Moreover, since labour is initiated by your baby producing certain hormones as he reaches full maturity, it follows that the actual date of delivery can vary fairly widely – even in "textbook" pregnancies.

WHEN LABOUR IS DELAYED

Doctors do become concerned if a pregnancy continues much beyond the estimated date of delivery because postmaturity and possible placental insufficiency pose risks to the health of your baby. The longer the baby continues to grow in the uterus, the larger he is likely to be, which will increase the chances of a difficult labour, and the possibility that the placenta will not be able to continue to support the baby over an extended period.

If you have a personal or maternal family history of longer than average pregnancies (43 or 44 weeks, for example), your doctor may be willing to allow you to go more than two weeks overdue without inducing labour – but your baby will be monitored in case problems develop.

Breech babies If you are only a week past your EDD, and your baby is still in the breech position, it may be an indication that he is not yet ready to be born because most babies do not usually stay in the head-down position until they are fully mature at about 37 weeks. Some babies remain breech until term.

Pelvic disproportion   Labour may be delayed if your baby's head is too big to pass through your pelvis. This disproportion may prevent the baby's head from becoming engaged and, if so, a Caesarean section is usually required.

POST-MATURE BABIES

An overdue baby is in danger of being post-mature. This means that your baby will have lost fat from all over his body, particularly his tummy. Consequently, his skin will look red and wrinkled as if it doesn't fit him, and it may have begun to peel. Very few babies are actually post-mature, but because post-maturity depends not only on the baby, but also on his placenta, it is difficult to predict which babies will be at risk.

What it means   The outcome of going well over your due date may include a longer and more difficult labour, because the post-mature baby tends to be bigger and the bones in his skull tend to be harder (which means that his descent through the birth canal is likely to be more traumatic both for him and for you). There is also an increased chance of stillbirth (the risk doubles by the 43rd week and triples by the 44th week). There is a further possibility that a uterus that seems to be slow to start labour may also be relatively inefficient during labour so that labour is unduly prolonged.

CHECKING THAT ALL IS WELL

Babies who have gone past their EDDs are monitored closely, and there are a number of different ways of keeping a check on your baby.

Fetal movement recording   One obvious sign that all is well with your baby is if you can detect regular fetal movements. Since all mothers and babies are different, the amount of movement that is normal for each individual pregnancy varies. You are the best judge of whether your unborn baby is acting normally, and you can monitor his activity by making a note of how many kicks you feel in a day.

Urinary oestriol tests These measure the amount of oestriol (a form of oestrogen) in your urine. The placenta produces oestriol in increasing amounts throughout pregnancy until just before labour begins, when oestriol production drops off. A lower oestriol level than might be expected suggests that the placenta is not functioning as well as it should. However, oestriol levels in your urine can vary by as much as 30 percent from day to day, even when everything is normal, so a series of readings will be taken.

Electronic fetal monitoring This may be used to check the baby's heartbeat before or during labour. A monitor is strapped around your abdomen. Using ultrasound, it provides a continuous sound or paper recording of the baby's heartbeat. If the heartbeat is satisfactory (particularly during a contraction, see below), doctors usually consider that it is unnecessary to perform other tests, or to induce labour.

Oxytocin test Oxytocin is the natural hormone that causes your uterus to contract, and is often used (in its synthetic form, Syntocinon) to induce labour. Occasionally, it is used to check on your baby's well-being.

For this test, a needle is inserted in your arm, and a small amount of Syntocinon is dripped in, which makes your uterus contract. The fetal heart is monitored throughout the contraction (when the baby's heart rate should slow down) and it is observed how quickly the heart rate returns to normal after the contraction. Any slowness in the return to a normal heart rate may indicate that the baby is distressed, and induction will almost certainly be advised.

CHAPTER 5

MEDICAL EMERGENCIES

If medical emergencies happen during pregnancy they tend to occur mainly in the first and third trimesters. In the first three months, the first trimester, most emergencies are associated with the loss of the fetus (miscarriage), or with it growing outside the uterus, as in an ectopic pregnancy. In the third trimester there may be complications such as pre-eclampsia, or problems with the placenta. These tend on the whole to be rare and most pregnancies are uneventful with the vast majority of babies being delivered safely. It is wise, however, to be aware of the danger signs so that you can seek medical help quickly if necessary.

VAGINAL
BLEEDING

Vaginal bleeding at any stage of pregnancy should be taken seriously. It may indicate an abnormally placed placenta, known as placenta praevia (see p. 70), or it may be a warning of imminent miscarriage. Both of these conditions require prompt medical treatment.

Vaginal bleeding occurs in the first trimester in about a quarter of all pregnancies. Over half of these pregnancies continue, with delivery of a healthy baby at term.

If at any time during your pregnancy vaginal bleeding occurs:

• *Call your doctor and go to bed at once.*

• *Lie flat with your legs and hips higher than your shoulders.*

• *If you pass any clots, mention this to your doctor, who may want to examine them.*

• *Don't take any medicine or drink any alcohol.*

EMERGENCY CONDITIONS

The vast majority of pregnancies continue to term with no problems or emergencies. However, it is sensible to make yourself aware of the danger signs so that you know when to seek professional medical attention.

MISCARRIAGE

Medically known as spontaneous abortion, miscarriage is when the fetus aborts before the 24th week. After the 24th week, it is called a stillbirth. About a third of all first pregnancies end in early miscarriage. A quarter occur before pregnancy has been diagnosed or even suspected, so women are often unaware that they have miscarried, believing that they have only had a period.

Miscarriage increases in frequency with age and with the number of previous pregnancies. They usually happen during the first trimester, the most common symptom being bleeding, which occurs in 95 percent of cases. If bleeding occurs at any time in your pregnancy, you must consult your doctor.

Most early miscarriages happen because the seriously abnormal fetus fails to implant securely in the uterine wall. Maternal causes of miscarriage include uterine abnormalities such as large fibroids and hormonal imbalances. Some bacterial and viral infections can also cause miscarriage. Cervical incompetence (see p. 72) accounts for only one percent of spontaneous abortions. Paternal factors include abnormal sperm and incompatible blood type that causes the mother to produce antibodies to her partner's blood. These antibodies then attack and kill her fetus. Doctors divide what we call miscarriage into several medical types:

Threatened abortion Miscarriage is possible but not inevitable. There is vaginal bleeding and sometimes pain. This occurs in about ten percent of all pregnancies and it may be confused with the slight bleeding that can occur at the time of the first missed period.

Inevitable abortion Vaginal bleeding is accompanied by pain because the uterus is contracting. Unfortunately, if there is also dilatation of the cervix, the loss of the embryo is bound to occur.

Complete abortion The fetus and placenta are expelled from the uterus, sometimes without any symptoms. This can be confirmed by ultrasound examination.

Missed abortion The fetus and placenta die, but remain in the uterus for some time, before being expelled. The symptoms of pregnancy disappear but there is no other indication of fetal death until later.

Incomplete abortion This is the term for when abortion has occurred but some of the products of conception, such as the amniotic sac or the placenta, remain in the uterus.

Habitual abortion Three or more miscarriages have occurred at the same stage of pregnancy, possibly for the same reason.

Recurrent abortion Miscarriage has occurred on three or more occasions, for different reasons and at different stages of pregnancy.

Treatment If you are bleeding, go to bed and stay there until the bleeding ceases. In particular, do not engage in activities such as strenuous exercise and sexual intercourse. If the bleeding and pain subside, you are quite likely to go on to deliver a healthy baby.

If miscarriage appears to be inevitable, there is little doctors can do to prevent it. Complete and incomplete abortions should always be treated in hospital. If an incomplete abortion occurs, the uterus will be cleaned out by a procedure called an ERPC (evacuation of retained products of conception) under general anaesthetic. Painkillers are given, along with drugs, to stop the bleeding. If a lot of blood has been lost (at least 500 millilitres/1 pint), a transfusion may be necessary.

There is no urgency in treating a missed abortion, but if, after a time, a spontaneous abortion hasn't occurred, an ERPC procedure will be carried out. If fetal death occurs later in pregnancy, prostaglandin pessaries or an oxytocin injection will be given to stimulate delivery.

Habitual abortion that has occurred because of cervical incompetence can be treated by running a "purse-string" suture round the cervix at the beginning of the next pregnancy to secure competency (see p. 72).

REASONS FOR REPEATED MISCARRIAGES

Possible reasons for frequent miscarriages (habitual abortion) include:

- *Genetic or hormonal disorders, which can often be pinpointed.*

- *Long-term infections, such as listeria, which may sometimes cause repeated miscarriages, and can be difficult to diagnose and treat.*

- *Poor nutrition.*

- *Chronic disease, such as renal disease.*

- *Cervical incompetence (see p. 72).*

- *Immune disorders, such as Rhesus blood incompatibility (see p. 62), in which the mother's immune system identifies the fetus as foreign, and attacks it. Suppressing the mother's immune reaction, or injecting the fetus with antibodies may be considered.*

- *Physical causes, including tumours in the uterus (particularly fibroids) or structural abnormalities such as a partial or complete septum, which is a partial or full partition of the uterus; these can usually be corrected by surgery.*

Even so, some mothers will repeatedly abort even though exhaustive tests reveal no specific cause. Recent research has shown that loving care can successfully heal this condition.

ABNORMAL POSITIONS OF THE PLACENTA

If the placenta has implanted incorrectly, it can obstruct the baby's birth.

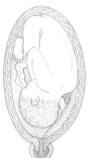

Side position
The placenta implants on the side and extends to the cervix, but does not cover it.

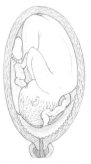

Blocking the cervix
The placenta implants centrally, completely covering the cervix – even when the cervix is fully dilated.

PLACENTAL SEPARATION

Bleeding can occur from the placental bed owing to partial or complete separation of the placenta from the uterus. Blood builds up in the spaces, and eventually escapes around the membranes and through the cervix into the vagina. Known as placental abruption (*abruptio placentae*), it occurs in about one in 200 pregnancies. The cause is unknown, but it tends to be more common in women who have had two or more children. Obstetricians divide placental separation into three types according to it's severity:

In *mild separation*, blood loss can be slight. Bed rest is the best treatment, with ultrasound examination to monitor the situation. If it occurs late in pregnancy, labour may be induced.

In *moderate separation*, a quarter of the placenta separates and 500 millilitres to one litre (between one and two pints) of blood are lost. This requires a blood transfusion and, if the baby is still alive, a Caesarean section is performed.

Severe separation is an acute emergency, when at least two-thirds of the placenta shears off the uterine wall, and up to two litres (four pints) of blood are lost. This causes severe shock, disturbance of blood coagulation, and full kidney shutdown. A rapid blood transfusion will be given, and if the pregnancy is approaching term, a Caesarean section will be performed to save the baby. If placental abruption occurs before the third trimester, fetal death is inevitable.

PLACENTA PRAEVIA

This occurs when the placenta is implanted in the lower segment of the uterus instead of the upper part (see column, left). It therefore lies in front of the baby when she has to descend the birth canal at the onset of labour. The baby cannot pass down the canal without dislodging the placenta, thereby interrupting her own blood supply. Placenta praevia is a major cause of bleeding after the 20th week and of haemorrhage in the final two months of pregnancy. The cause is usually unknown.

The greater the proportion of the placenta lying in the lower uterine segment, the greater the likelihood of complications during delivery. Even though the growth of the placenta slows down after the 30th week of pregnancy, the lower segment of the uterus is increasing in length. Stresses between the placenta and the uterine wall may occur, leading to episodes of bleeding.

This extremely dangerous condition can be diagnosed well ahead of delivery by ultrasound scan (see p. 32). Early symptoms include episodes of bleeding, with bright red blood, which may occur after sexual intercourse. If this happens, the doctor will advise hospital admission for bed rest, with a blood transfusion if necessary. Bed rest should continue, if possible, until the 37th week, when the baby will be delivered by Caesarean section.

Postpartum haemorrhage is likely to occur after the delivery of the baby and drugs to prevent it will be given as soon as the baby is born. In a very few cases, haemorrhage will continue despite treatment and then a hysterectomy may have to be considered. For these reasons, delivery in a well-equipped hospital where a blood transfusion service is on hand is vital.

PLACENTAL INSUFFICIENCY

During pregnancy, the fetus receives oxygen and nourishment and excretes carbon dioxide and waste products via the umbilical cord and the placenta. A healthy placenta, which is one that is able to act as an effective organ of transfer for the entire pregnancy, is therefore crucial in maintaining the health of the fetus.

Assessment and treatment Insufficiency may be indicated if you show less than normal weight gain, if your uterus is growing too slowly, or if your baby's development is below normal.

Ultrasound is the most reliable way to measure the growth of the baby. If it shows that the baby is not growing adequately, your doctor will carry out tests that measure placental hormone and enzyme levels in the blood. A bio-physical profile that takes account of fetal breathing, body movement, tone and quantity of amniotic fluid may also be compiled. A specialized ultrasound scan called a Doppler scan (see p. 34) has now been developed; this can tell doctors about the flow of blood through the placenta, indicating whether it is working properly. Placental insufficiency may warrant the induction of labour and possibly a Caesarean section.

REASONS FOR PLACENTAL INSUFFICIENCY

The placenta may be unable to support the fetus adequately for a number of reasons:

- *The placenta may have developed abnormally.*

- *Blood flow through the placenta may be restricted, or placental tissue lost because of a blood clot.*

- *The placenta may separate, or partly separate, from the uterine wall.*

- *The placenta may be too small or poorly developed.*

- *The pregnancy may go beyond dates, so that the ageing placenta becomes inadequate for the fetus.*

- *If the mother has diabetes, this can affect the placenta adversely.*

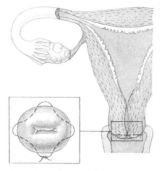

Suturing the cervix
The cervix is kept closed by passing a suture right around it – like the strings of a purse. The thread is normally cut about seven days before the expected date of delivery.

INCOMPETENT CERVIX

During pregnancy, the cervix normally remains tightly shut and is sealed with a plug of mucus. This means that the fetus is safely held in the uterus until labour begins, when the cervix begins to dilate. Occasionally, however, the cervical canal is incompetent and begins to open before term, usually in the third or fourth month. This allows the amniotic sac containing the fetus to sag through into the vagina, and possibly rupture, with a sudden loss of amniotic fluid followed by miscarriage. Unless the cervix has been damaged during previous surgery or pregnancy, this condition is fortunately rare. However, an incompetent cervix is usually diagnosed only after a first miscarriage has occurred.

If cervical incompetence is thought to be the cause of a previous miscarriage, treatment involves suturing your cervix, which means a soft non-absorbable thread is inserted in the cervix to keep it closed (see column, left). The thread is cut approximately seven days before term, and your baby is delivered vaginally in the normal way.

PRE-ECLAMPSIA

Pregnancy-induced hypertension (high blood pressure), or pre-eclampsia, is a potentially dangerous condition that can affect as many as one in ten women, especially first-time mothers and women carrying more than one baby. It is unique to pregnancy, starting at any time in the second half. It is not known what causes it, but it does tend to run in families. We do know that pre-eclampsia arises in the placenta and so the baby may grow more slowly than normal.

Symptoms Pre-eclampsia is symptomless, but raised blood pressure and protein in the urine detected at an antenatal visit may alert staff to its presence.

Treatment A pregnancy complicated by pre-eclampsia cannot be restored to normal, but delivery of the baby and placenta ends the disease. Admission to hospital allows close monitoring of mother and baby so that delivery can be arranged before serious complications such as eclampsia (see below) arise. For almost every mother, delivery of the baby reverses all the effects.

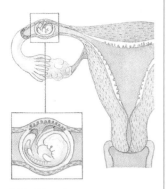

Tubal implantation
Ectopic pregnancy occurs in about 1 in every 300 pregnancies. The egg usually implants in the Fallopian tube (99%). Very rarely, it may implant elsewhere.

ECLAMPSIA

The word eclampsia derives from the Greek words meaning "like a flash of lightening" because it seemed to strike out of the blue with fits and, eventually, coma. Eclampsia is a potentially life-threatening condition for both mother and baby and it used to be quite common. However, it is now extremely rare in the West owing to the ability of doctors to diagnose the condition in its earliest phase (pre-eclampsia, see opposite) and doctors and midwives are constantly alert for the warning signs. When eclampsia does occur, it is a full-blown medical emergency.

Symptoms Eclampsia is an emergency because the blood vessels in the uterus go into spasm (vasospasm), thereby cutting down the blood flow to the fetus with dangerous tissue hypoxia (low oxygen).

The mother's life is threatened because vasospasm leads to kidney failure. Brain oxygen is also lowered, causing heightened brain sensitivity, which shows as fits. Tissues become waterlogged because of fluid retention and haemorrhages can occur in tissues such as the liver. The earliest signs are drowsiness, headache, dimness of vision, all of which are superimposed on rising blood pressure, swelling of hands, face and feet (oedema), and protein in the urine.

Treatment Where eclampsia develops, like pre-eclampsia (see opposite) treatment is aimed at delivering the baby, increasing blood flow to the brain and reducing high blood pressure – usually by Caesarean section. As soon as the baby is delivered the condition subsides.

ECTOPIC PREGNANCY

In ectopic pregnancy, the fertilized egg implants somewhere other than in the cavity of the uterus, usually in a Fallopian tube (see column, left). The rapidly growing embryo causes the tube to distend, and the invading placenta weakens its walls, causing bleeding. Eventually the tube bursts under the strain.

However, before this, certain symptoms that signal all is not well (see column, right) usually occur around the sixth week of pregnancy. Report these to your doctor at once.

TYPES OF ECTOPIC PREGNANCY

Doctors define two forms of ectopic pregnancy:

Subacute *This is signalled by pain in the abdomen, usually only on one side, sometimes with vaginal bleeding, fainting and pain in the shoulder (on the same side as the pain in the abdomen). It may not be detected until eight to ten weeks' gestation. It is sometimes treatable by injecting a drug into the embryo, causing it to die and be reabsorbed, which can save the Fallopian tube.*

Acute form *This happens when the tube bursts, leading to severe pain and shock and falling blood pressure. A ruptured ectopic pregnancy is a surgical emergency and requires immediate hospital admission and treatment by surgical removal of the pregnancy from the Fallopian tube.*

PATERNITY LEAVE

In Britain and the US there is no provision in law for paid paternity leave. In practice, most fathers take some time off around the birth of a child either as unpaid leave or as part of their paid leave entitlement.

Trade unions and enlightened employers are gradually recognizing the importance of this time and are beginning to include paternity leave in their contracts.

In Scandinavian countries fathers receive pay while taking paternity leave, which means that nearly all fathers take it, to the benefit of all concerned.

RETURNING TO WORK

It is the law in Great Britain that your job must be kept open for you from 11 weeks prior to your expected date of delivery until 28 weeks after the birth, provided that you have been with your employer for two years' full-time or five years' part-time, and you work until the 29th week of your pregnancy.

Discuss these conditions with your employer and make it clear that you wish to return to work so that your job will be kept open for you. Your employer may have more generous maternity pay and leave entitlements than those provided by law.

YOUR RIGHTS

Pregnant women are entitled to certain rights and benefits depending on their circumstances and national insurance contributions. The entitlements, particularly for those on low incomes, are complicated but any Social Security office or Citizens Advice Bureau will be able to work out what you can claim for. If you are employed, ask your employer or your trade union representative about your maternity leave and pay.

STATE BENEFITS

The Maternity Allowance is a tax-free allowance you may receive if you can't get Statutory Maternity Pay (see below) because you have recently stopped working, changed jobs or become self-employed. It is paid for a maximum of 18 weeks and is dependent on your national insurance contributions.

If you or your partner are receiving Income Support, Jobseeker's Allowance, Family Credit or Disability Allowance, you may be able to get a cash payment (called a Maternity Payment) from the Social Fund. The rules are explained in leaflets that you can get from your local Social Security office, Citizens Advice Bureau or antenatal clinic.

During your pregnancy and for one year after the birth you are also eligible for free prescriptions and dental treatment, and you may get free milk if you are on a low income.

WORKING WOMEN

If you are an employee, you are entitled to 14 weeks' maternity leave. If you have been in continuous work with your employer for more than two years (full-time), you are entitled to a further 26 weeks maternity leave. For the first six weeks of maternity leave you receive pay at 90 percent of your average weekly earnings, followed by 12 weeks at Statutory Maternity Pay rate. If you have been employed for less than two years, you get only the latter. You don't have to be intending to return to work to receive these payments. The government refunds the money to your employer. You are also entitled to time off with pay to attend your antenatal clinic and classes and you are protected against unfair dismissal when pregnant.

WORK HAZARDS

If your job is dangerous or it would be illegal for you to continue doing it, for example, if you work with anaesthetic gases or toxic chemicals, your employer must find you an alternative job or transfer you to a non-hazardous working place.

Claiming Your Rights
The chart below gives you a timetable for claiming benefits and notifying your employer, so that you can be sure of getting your maximum entitlement in terms of money and rights.

RIGHTS AND BENEFITS TIMETABLE

WHEN	WHAT TO DO	WHY
As soon as you know you are pregnant.	1 Ask doctor or midwife for form FW8. 2 Tell your dentist (if you need treatment). 3 Check leaflet HC11 and tell Social Security office if getting Income Support. 4 Tell your employer. 5 Find out if you can get Maternity Allowance.	1 To apply for free prescriptions. 2 To apply for free dental treatment. 3 To check your right to free spectacles. and help with hospital fares. 4 To check if you can get SMP (Statutory Maternity Pay); for right to paid time off for antenatal visits. 5 If you can't get SMP.
As soon as you can.	If you are unemployed or sick, check with Social Security office about Maternity Allowance claim.	It can affect the amount of Maternity Allowance you may get.
At least 3 weeks before you intend to stop working.	Tell your employer in writing: the date you will stop working, when the baby is due, and whether you intend to return to your job.	To protect your rights to SMP, and to return to work.
As soon after the birth as you can.	1 If baby was late, fill in form BM9. 2 Register baby's birth. 3 Send off form for Child Benefit and Family Premium if you are a single parent. 4 Check low income benefits.	1 To claim extra Maternity Allowance. 2 To get the birth certificate. 3 To get Child Benefit and Lone Parent payment. 4 To see if you qualify for Maternity Payment from Social Fund, and spectacles, milk and vitamins, hospital fares and help with your rent and council tax.
3 weeks after birth or 6 weeks after birth.	Register baby (if you live in Scotland). Register baby (places other than Scotland).	Latest date to do this. Latest date to do this.
3 weeks before returning to work.	Write to your employer stating the date that you wish to return.	To protect your right to return to work.
When the baby is 28 weeks old.	Latest date by which you have a right to go back to your job.	You may lose your right to return to work.

USEFUL ADDRESSES

Active Birth Centre
Bickerton House,
25 Bickerton Road,
London N19 5JT
Tel: 0171 561 9006

Information and classes on active involvement in childbirth at home or in hospital

Acumedic
101–105 Camden High Street,
London NW1 7JN
Tel: 0171 388 5783/6704

For the hire of a TENS (Transcutaneous Electrical Nerve Stimulation) machine

AIMS (Association for Improvements in Maternity Services)
40 Kingswood Avenue,
London NW6 6LS
Tel: 0181 960 5585

Pressure group that campaigns for the right of parents to have the maternity services they want

APEC (Action on Pre-eclampsia)
31–33 College Road,
Harrow, Middlesex HA1 1EJ
Tel: 01923 266778

Aqua Birth Pools
Active Birth Centre,
Bickerton House,
25 Bickerton Road,
London N19 5JT
Tel: 0171 561 9006

For the hire of a portable water birth pool

Association of Breastfeeding Mothers
PO Box 441,
St Albans
Herts AL4 0AS
Tel: 0181 778 4769

A 24-hour telephone service for mothers. Supplies nationwide network of breastfeeding counsellors

Association for Postnatal Illness
25 Jerdan Place,
London SW6 1BE
Tel: 0171 386 0868

Advice to on how to cope with postnatal depression

Bereavement groups
(for parents whose babies die in special care) see SANDS opposite.

Birthworks
Unit 3F,
Brent Mill Trading Estate,
South Brent, Devon TQ10 9YT
Tel: 01364 72802

Advice and literature on water births, birth pools for hire

BLISSLINK
17–21 Emerald Street,
London WC1N 3QL
Freephone: 0500 151617

Advice and support for parents with special-care babies

British Acupuncture Council
Park House,
206–208 Latimer Road,
London W2 6RE
Tel: 0181 964 0222

British Diabetic Association
10 Queen Anne Street,
London W1M 0BD
Tel: 0171 323 1531

Advice for pregnant women with diabetes

British Epilepsy Association
Anstey House,
40 Hanover Square,
Leeds LS3 1BE
Tel: 01132 439393

British Homeopathy Association
27a Devonshire Street,
London W1N 1RJ
Tel: 0171 935 2163

Caesarean Support Network
55 Cooil Drive,
Douglas, Isle of Man
Tel: 01254 661269 (after 6 pm)

Chelsea and Westminster Hospital
369 Fulham Road,
London SW10
Tel: 0181 746 8000

Contact for birth plan information and charts

Down's Syndrome Association
155 Mitcham Road,
London SW17 9PG
Tel: 0181 682 4001

Advice on the care of children with Down's syndrome

Federation of Recruitment and Employment Services
36–38 Mortimer Street,
London W1N 7RB
Tel: 0171 323 4300

Provides a list of nanny and au pair agencies; send SAE for information

Foresight
28 The Paddock,
Godalming,
Surrey GU7 1XD
Tel: 01483 427839

Pre-pregnancy advice and consultation on infertility and miscarriage; send SAE for further information

Freeline Social Security Number
0800 666555

Free helpline for information about maternity benefits

Gingerbread
16–17 Clerkenwell Close,
London EC1R 0AA
Tel: 0171 336 8183

A mutual support group for one-parent families

Independent Midwives' Association
94 Auckland Road,
London SE19 2DB
Tel: 0181 406 3172

Network of independent midwives offering private care

La Leche League
PO Box BM 3424,
London WC1N 3XX
Tel: 0171 242 1278

Advice and information about breastfeeding

MAMA (Meet-a-Mum Association)
Cornerstone House,
14 Willis Road,
Croydon CR0 2XX
Tel: 0181 665 0357

Help for new parents, especially mothers with postnatal depression

Maternity Alliance
45 Beech Street,
London EC2P 2AX
Tel: 0171 588 8582

Information on maternity rights and benefits

Miscarriage Association
c/o Claytoll Hospital,
Northgate, Wakefield,
West Yorkshire WF1 3JS
Tel: 01924 200799

Information on a network of miscarriage support groups

MS Therapy Centres
Bradbury House,
155 Barkers Lane,
Bedford MK41 9RX
Tel: 01234 325781

Information for pregnant women suffering from MS

National Childbirth Trust
Alexandra House,
Oldham Terrace, Acton,
London W3 6NH
Tel: 0181 992 8637

Nationwide antenatal classes and practical postnatal help

National Childminding Association
8 Masons Hill,
Bromley,
Kent BR2 9EY
Tel: 0181 464 6164

National Council for One-Parent Families
255 Kentish Town Road,
London NW5 2LX
Tel: 0171 428 5400

Advice and referral service for one-parent families

PAL (Parents [London] Anonymous)
6 Manor Gardens,
London N7 6LA
Tel: 0171 263 8918

A 24-hour helpline for parents who are under stress

RCOG (Royal College of Obstetricians and Gynaecologists)
27 Sussex Place,
Regent's Park,
London NW1 4RG
Tel: 0171 262 5425

Helpline and leaflets

Royal College of Midwives
15 Mansfield Street,
London W1M 0BE
Tel: 0171 580 6523/4/5

St Mary's Hospital Recurrent Miscarriage Clinic
Winston Churchill Wing,
Praed Street,
London W2 1NY
Tel: 0171 258 0285

SANDS (Stillbirth and Neonatal Death Society),
28 Portland Place,
London W1N 4DE
Tel: 0171 436 5881

National support network for bereaved parents

Splashdown Waterbirth Services
17 Wellington Terrace,
Harrow-on-the-Hill,
Middlesex HA1 3EP
Tel: 0181 422 9308

Birth pools for hire

TAMBA (Twins and Multiple Birth Association)
PO Box 30, Little Sutton,
South Wirral L66 1TH
Tel: 0151 348 0020

Offers encouragement and support for parents before and after multiple births

Vegetarian Society
Parkdale, Dunham Road,
Altrincham,
Cheshire WA14 4QG
Tel: 0161 928 0793

Nutritional advice for pregnant women who are vegetarians

Women's Health
52 Featherstone Street,
London EC1Y 8RT
Tel: 0171 251 6580

Advice on reproductive health

INDEX

ACKNOWLEDGMENTS

Dorling Kindersley would like to thank the following individuals and organizations for their contributions to this book.

PHOTOGRAPHY
All photographs by Ranald Mackechnie except Howard Sochurek/Hillelson page 33.

MEDICAL CONSULTANTS
Gwen Atwood; Leonora Branski; Dr. Nigel Brown; Dr. Felicity Challoner; Prof. Geoffrey Chamberlain; The Hallam Medical Centre; Dr. Kypros Nicolaides; Prof. Cheryl Tickle; Dr. Robert Whittle.

EQUIPMENT
Mothercare UK Ltd – maternity and baby clothes; equipment; and toys.

INDEX
Hilary Bird

TEXT FILM OUTPUT
The Brightside Partnership, London